Dr. Alan H. Pressm ... **rd** ceritified dietitian/nutritionist . He is the former chairman of the Department of Clinical Nutrition at New York Chiropractic College and served numerous terms as president for the Council on Nutrition of the American Chiropractic Association. He is also a diplomate and past president of the American Chiropractic Board of Nutrition.

Dr. Pressman has been a regular contributor on CNBC, and is a noted veteran radio guest on ABC and WOR talk radio. His expertise on a wide range of topical health issues has been heard by millions on the nationally syndicated radio show, *Dr. Pressman on Health* on WEVD (10.50 AM-NY). He is currently the director of Gramercy Health Associates in New York City.

Herbert D. Goodman, M.D., Ph.D., F.A.D.E.P., is a noted medical practitioner of both traditional and alternative medicine. His specialties include emergency medicine, pain management, acupuncture, geriatrics, and hypnosis.

Dr. Goodman is a Fellow in the American Academy of Disability Evaluating Physicians, a diplomate in the American Academy of Pain Management, and was elected as an approved consultant for the American Society of Clinical Hypnosis. He is currently director of the Southwestern Center for Pain in Phoenix, Arizona.

DON'T MISS THE OTHER BOOKS IN
THE PHYSICIANS' GUIDES SERIES

Treating Arthritis, Carpal Tunnel Syndrome, and Joint Conditions
Treating Hypertension and Other Cardiovascular Conditions
Treating Gynecological Conditions
Treating Digestive Conditions

Coming soon from Berkley Books

THE PHYSICIANS' GUIDES TO HEALING

TREATING ASTHMA, ALLERGIES, AND FOOD SENSITIVITIES

Alan Pressman, D.C., Ph.D., D.A.C.B.N., C.C.N., and Herbert D. Goodman, M.D., Ph.D., with Rachelle Bernadette Nones

Developed by The Philip Lief Group, Inc.

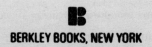

BERKLEY BOOKS, NEW YORK

This book is meant to educate and should not be used as an alternative to proper medical care. No treatments mentioned herein should be taken without qualified medical consultation and approval. The authors have exerted every effort to ensure that the information presented is accurate up to the time of publication. However, in light of ongoing research and the constant flow of information, it is possible that new findings may invalidate some of the data presented here.

TREATING ASTHMA, ALLERGIES, AND FOOD SENSITIVITIES

A Berkley Book / published by arrangement with
The Philip Lief Group, Inc.

PRINTING HISTORY
Berkley edition / April 1997

All rights reserved.
Copyright © 1997 by The Philip Lief Group, Inc.
Cover illustration by Arthur Gager.
This book may not be reproduced in whole or in part,
by mimeograph or any other means, without permission.
For information address: The Berkley Publishing Group,
200 Madison Avenue, New York, New York 10016.

The Putnam Berkley World Wide Web site address is
http://www.berkley.com/berkley

ISBN: 0-425-15669-9

BERKLEY®
Berkley Books are published by The Berkley Publishing Group,
200 Madison Avenue, New York, New York 10016.
BERKLEY and the "B" design
are trademarks belonging to Berkley Publishing Corporation.

PRINTED IN THE UNITED STATES OF AMERICA

10 9 8 7 6 5 4 3 2 1

Contents

Introduction

ARE YOU HEALTHY?

The answer to the above question may depend upon whom you ask. Allopathic medicine, also called conventional, traditional, or Western medicine, defines health as the absence of disease. In the allopathic approach, chemical medications and surgical operations are the primary tools of healing. Much of the power to heal relies upon the progress of modern technology for its theories and practices. By contrast, holistic—also called alternative or natural—medicine is based on preventive care and focuses not only on bodily health but on psychological and spiritual health as well. To the holistic practitioner, good health is as much a reflection of our lifestyle and emotional stability as it is a product of our avoiding disease and eating the proper foods. In the holistic vision of wellness, a balanced union of physical, spiritual, and emotional states produces vibrancy and longevity.

Clearly, allopathic and holistic practitioners approach health care from different vantage points. But there has been a revolution within the traditional medical establishment, and a new era has begun—one that integrates alternative therapy and theories of overall wellness with allopathic medicine, its rigorous practices of surgery and use of pharmaceuticals. Also known as complementary medicine, the fusion of the two schools of medicine has become the new frontier of health care. At last, patients can benefit from the collective wisdom of both ideologies of medical thought.

The *Physicians' Guides to Healing* series has been developed to give readers insight into the benefits of complementary medicine on a variety of health issues. The series consists of five authoritative health reference books, each of which provides accurate and up-to-date information on treatments from the perspectives of allopathic, alternative, and complementary medicine. The titles in the series—*Treating Asthma, Allergies, and Food Sensitivities; Treating Arthritis, Carpal Tunnel Syndrome, and Joint Conditions; Treating Hypertension and Other Cardiovascular Conditions; Treating Gynecological Conditions;* and *Treating Digestive Conditions*—will help the reader understand and compare both allopathic and alternative approaches to specific health problems, and make informed decisions about which combination of therapies is best suited to individual needs.

Dr. Herbert Goodman and Dr. Alan Pressman, coauthors of the series, lend their unsurpassed medical expertise to each volume. Both practitioners incorporate elements of natural medicine into their own traditional practices, approaching their patients' needs in a broad-minded and sensitive manner. Each book in the series reflects their confidence in complementary medicine and includes several case studies that closely examine the health problems and genuine concerns of real people. These case histories demonstrate the potential healing power of complementary therapy when all else has failed, and they show how a candid and trusting relationship between doctor and patient is essential to effective and precise treatment.

Although the goals of both allopathic and alternative

medicine are similar—health, immunity to diseases, and well-being—the approaches of holistic care focus more on preparing the body for a lifetime of total body health through healthy living, natural healing, and overall wellness rather than on curing specific illnesses as they arise. The various areas of alternative medicine include: mind/body control, as displayed in studies of art, dance, music therapy, biofeedback, yoga, and psychotherapy; manual healing therapies, such as acupressure, Alexander technique, chiropractic, massage, osteopathy, reflexology, and therapeutic touch; bioelectromagnetic therapy involving techniques such as blue light, artificial lighting, electrostimulation, and neuromagnetic stimulation; diet and nutrition, including vitamins, nutritional supplements, and practices like Gerson therapy; and herbal medicine, among other options. These are a few of the holistic remedies that you will become familiar with as you read the *Physicians' Guides to Healing*.

Of course, traditional treatments offer just as wide a range of possibilities and countless benefits. For instance, without the technology of modern surgical procedures and the mechanics of pacemakers, many people who suffer from irregular heartbeats would not be able to survive; likewise, without specialists' knowledge of orthopedic reconstruction operations, torn ligaments and deteriorated cartilage would prevent many injured people from walking. Cancerous tumors, including breast cancer, might claim the lives of thousands of cancer patients were it not for allopathic procedures such as mastectomies. Millions of cancer patients have extended their lives and improved their chances of survival with treatments such as surgery, radiation, and chemotherapy.

TRADITIONAL MEDICINE: A BRIEF HISTORY

Our knowledge of traditional medicine dates back as far as written history, although prescientific healing practices were based on magic, talismans, spells, incantations, and folk remedies ("old wives' tales"). Rudimentary surgery from the days before scientific medicine involved procedures such as trepanning, which entailed boring holes in the skull to relieve headaches, insanity, and epilepsy. As early as the third century B.C., doctors gained status as scientists, distinct from sorcerers and priests. Egyptian doctors are reported to have been trained for their profession by learning the arts of interrogation, inspection, and palpation (examination by touch). The drugs available to the Egyptians, though primitive, are still in use today, including figs, dates, and castor oil for laxative purposes, and tannic acid to soothe and treat burns. Early Mesopotamians also discovered a wealth of primitive pharmaceuticals in various forms, many of which were derived from mineral sources. The Mesopotamians are renowned for being the first society to develop accurate models of the liver which they regarded as "the seat of the soul." This was the dawn of pharmacology, anatomy, and physiology.

The teachings of Hippocrates, the "father of medicine" who lived in Greece during the third century B.C., are the foundation of the modern medical values. His Hippocratic oath, which established a code of medical honor, is a vow of integrity that people in the health care industry take even today. Herophilus, an Egyptian from the same time period, is reported to have performed the first public dissection of a human cadaver. The founder of comparative anatomy was the Greek philosopher Aristotle, who also publicly performed dissections of many animals. According to etched records, early Egyptians performed castrations, removal of bladder stones, amputations, and various optical surgeries. Hindus in the second and third centuries A.D. performed the first known plastic surgery by grafting skin from the thigh and buttocks onto the nose. Chinese drugs in the same period included rhubarb, aconite, sulfur, animal organs, and—most importantly—opium, a powerful and effective pain reliever and anesthetic. The interest in the human body, the study of various types of life forms, and these early attempts at surgery and remedial drug use provided the foundations for the rest of medical evolution.

The Middle Ages in Europe were times of scientific advances as more empirical and physical knowledge accumulated among learned men. The Italians were the first people to officially separate science from religion in the ninth and tenth centuries, allowing progress to be propelled by research and analysis—not faith. In the thirteenth century, several countries, including France and Italy, saw the formation of the medieval guilds, which were social-class rankings based upon profession. Barbers had always performed elementary surgery until the establishment of guilds. At that point, surgeons gained increased training, respect, and social status while barbers resigned themselves to haircutting and beard-shaving. In 1543, the publication of a treatise called *On the Structure of the Human Body* by the Belgian anatomist Andreas Vesalius prompted a surge in medical research and the development of new physiological discoveries. In the same decade, colleagues and students of Vesalius made the first diagnoses of ear diseases and the identification of fallopian tubes, eye muscles, tear ducts, and they arrived at the notion of a circulatory system.

The most important milestone in seventeenth-century medicine was the discovery by English physician William Harvey

of the exact mechanism of blood circulation, a discovery that
incited closer studies of the heart, lungs, and lymph systems
as well. The introduction of quinine—a drug used to treat tuberculosis patients—was another major event in therapeutic
progress during the seventeenth century. During this same
period, French physician Ambroise Paré was nicknamed
"the father of modern surgery" because he discovered that
ligating arteries with a red-hot iron could be used to control
bleeding and increase the patient's chances for survival.
This discovery enabled doctors to perform surgery without
worrying about time constraints or their patients' deaths
from blood loss.

The notion of germs was taken quite seriously by nine-
teenth-century medical practitioners, and the use of carbolic
acid (believed to kill germs) became a reliable way to reduce the likelihood of wound infections. Contributions to
the understanding of shock management and antibiotic administration also greatly increased success rates in surgery.
Other contributions from this century include X rays, discovered accidentally by Dr. Wilhelm Conrad Röntgen in
Germany, and the use of ultraviolet radiation for treating
many skin diseases, including psoriasis and tuberculosis of
the skin. American scientists contributed significant research and understanding to operative gynecology: in 1809,
Ephraim McDowell of Kentucky performed the first successful removal of an ovarian tumor, marking the dawn of
modern surgical procedure in the United States. Although
medicine was rapidly achieving new and amazing goals,
there were inevitable failures. For example, in the eighteenth century, John Brown promoted the theory that disease
was caused by a lack of stimulation, and he therefore pro-
posed stimulating his patients into health by bombarding
them with "heroic" doses of poisonous drugs like mercuric

chloride. Needless to say, not all of Dr. Brown's remedies resulted in restoring vigor and health to his patients.

The development of new ideas and technologies in the twentieth century has exponentially increased the magnitude of physical, chemical, surgical, and pharmacological knowledge. In addition to contributing to a general improvement in living conditions and a greater awareness of health issues, science has progressed into the realms of the previously inconceivable and impossible. For example, in the field of genetics, DNA replication is now possible; ultrasound technology makes viewing the fetus a normal prenatal procedure; and human life is readily created outside the woman's body by means of *in vitro* fertilization. And who would have believed that body parts could be reattached to the body, enabling dead tissue to come back to life? In 1962, the first successful limb replacement was performed: an arm, completely severed at the shoulder, was rejoined. Synthetic materials now allow surgeons to perform surgical replacements of hips, arms, teeth, and so on. Additionally, kidney and other organ transplants are now routinely successful.

Infectious diseases are largely under control now that most people have access to improved antibiotics, vaccines, and sanitation. The "wonder drugs" of the nineteenth and twentieth centuries have virtually wiped out most major diseases: sulfonamide antibiotics treat syphilis; streptomycin kills tuberculosis; sulfones treat leprosy; quinine treats malaria. Vaccines were developed for almost all of the most epidemic-threatening diseases: for smallpox (1796), typhoid fever (1897), diphtheria (1923), tetanus (1930s), and for yellow fever, measles, mumps, and rubella. The discovery of penicillin in 1938 by Englishmen Howard Florey and Ernst Chain vastly reduced World War II fatalities and continues to effectively treat many types of infections. Genetic engineering, a concept that originated in the 1980s, led to the development of vaccines for herpes simplex, hepatitis B, influenza, and chicken pox. In general, scientists and physicians now have a vastly improved understanding of the human body's immune system and can therefore anticipate and eliminate most significant health hazards. Even with modern-day health horrors such as AIDS, the Ebola virus, and increased cancer incidence rates, we can have faith that science will eventually find more and better treatments for such diseases.

Cardiovascular disease, one of the most threatening contemporary medical conditions, has recently become less of an enigma thanks to imaging techniques like magnetic resonance imaging (MRI) developed in the 1970s. Cardiac catheterization, which enables measurements of pressure to be taken in the heart, helps doctors analyze potential heart conditions. Also, an array of drugs—including chemicals that have been developed to block certain functions of the sympathetic nervous system—is now available to treat angina, heart arrhythmia, and hypertension. Bypass surgery (replacing arteries damaged or narrowed by cholesterol buildup) and the transplantation of temporary and permanent artificial hearts have greatly widened options for sufferers of cardiovascular conditions. Such inventions and discoveries, complemented with essential nutritional information on reducing cholesterol, sodium, and fat intake, make controlling cardiovascular risk factors easier.

The new horizons in modern medicine promise a wealth of possibilities. Some practices that are now in their incipient stages with great promises for the future include cryogenics (freezing blood in surgeries such as those for Parkinson's disease and for brain tumors), psychopharmacology (which has virtually replaced the barbaric practice of prefrontal lobotomy), microsurgery (used, for example, to operate on the inner ear), the use of plastics (silicon and Teflon) to replace defective body parts, and transplantation (of teeth, livers, hearts, endocrine glands).

Modern medicine has evolved considerably since the days of trepanning, bloodletting with leeches, and induced purgation with mercuric chloride. Allopathic practitioners have begun to incorporate holistic therapies into their treatment programs, and they have accepted many of the ideas that were once only acknowledged by alternative practitioners, some of which are described below. The result: a progressive, preventive approach to healing, and the widely accepted conviction that complementary medicine works wonders. In 1992 the federal government established the Office of Alternative Medicine as part of the National Institutes of Health (NIM)—conclusive proof that alternative medicine has indeed entered the mainstream.

ALTERNATIVE MEDICINE: A BRIEF HISTORY

Natural medicine has always existed in various manifestations. Even before the advent of technological innovations and chemical research, human beings have taken the steps necessary to restore good health by using any remedy that appeared to positively affect their ailments. Long before modern pain medicine, Native Americans chewed on willow bark to relieve pain and headaches. Nowadays people are more likely to reach for a couple of aspirin tablets, but the principle is the same: willow contains salicylic acid, the same ingredient used to produce aspirin. We all want to drink ginger ale when we're feeling sick, but do you know the reason why? The properties of the herbal ginger root are known to settle stomachaches. Even if carbonated ginger ale hasn't been around for centuries, ginger tonic certainly has. The principles of natural healing have inspired many non-invasive cures for pain and illness throughout history. Throughout history, Eastern medicine has been particularly successful in finding natural cures and using the body's inherent ability to heal itself from within. Much of what we consider "alternative" is simply Eastern in origin.

One of the oldest recorded alternative treatments is acupuncture, which dates back to 2000 B.C. Chinese healers developed acupuncture in response to the theory that there are special points known as meridians on the body connected to the internal organs and that vital energy flows along the lines that connect the meridians. According to this theory, diseases are caused by interruptions in the energy flow; inserting and twirling acupuncture needles into certain meridian points can stimulate energy and restore the body's normal energy flow. Acupuncture is widely used today in most Chinese hospitals for relieving pain, but only about ten percent of American practitioners have recognized its efficacy and use it to treat patients. It is used as an analgesic for a wide variety of problems and is commonly employed in the treatment of brain surgery, ulcers, hypertension, asthma, and various heart conditions. The modern, physiological explanation for why and how acupuncture works, according to American neurophysiologists, is based on the theory that endorphins and enkephalins (the body's natural pain killers) are released when the skin is pierced by needles.

In the late eighteenth century, in defiance of the common medical procedure resulting from theories such as Dr. Brown's, Samuel Hahneman devised a theory that "likes are cured by likes," meaning that the body's natural defenses could be implemented to cure any ailment with the help of natural, botanical stimulants. Hahneman's theory was the birth of homeopathy as we know it today. His idea of using the elements already available to us in nature (such as chamomile flowers or Kombucha mushrooms) and within our own bodies (such as our highly complex and effective immune system) gave birth to a set of practices that continues to generate innovative techniques for holistic healing today. Homeopathy was introduced to the United States in 1825, and the American Institute of Homeopathy was founded in 1844.

An important milestone in the development of holistic medicine was the emergence of naturopathy, which means "natural curing." In 1902 a German doctor named Benedict Lust brought his theory of naturopathy to America. He had been impressed by the benefits he had witnessed in Europe when people who visited water spas would return refreshed, relaxed, and invigorated. He recognized that nature's abundant natural resources—like water and sun—could be tapped and utilized as great healing agents. Water curing has always been an effective therapeutic treatment; just think of relaxing in a hot tub or taking a long hot shower to unwind after a stressful day of work. The term *hydrotherapy* was coined shortly after Hahneman imported the idea to America. In some European countries today, a visit to the health spa for a water cure is covered by health insurance. Dr. Lust is responsible for a wider acceptance of natural medicine during his time than in any other period in modern medicine, present-day excluded. He also believed in preventive measures such as good diet, exercise, mud baths, chiropractic massage, and other natural treatments. These fundamental tenets, along with Samuel Hahneman's, are still the cornerstones of holistic medicine today.

The major advancement of health care technology, especially in areas of surgery and pharmacology in the 1930s, is responsible for some of the deep segregation between homeopathic and traditional medicine. Earlier this century, there was virtually no way for homeopaths to spread the good word about such practices as hydrotherapy, botanical herbal treatments, or the benefits of massage—especially in the face of impressive medical and chemical breakthroughs in allopathic medicine. Chemical and drug companies had—and continue to have—a major financial stake in the promotion of allopathic medications and treatments; as a result, natural remedies have been brushed aside in a storm of advertising and promotion on the part of those larger drug companies and the allopathic practitioners who have advocated them.

Even the earliest homeopaths recognized the importance of regulating one's lifestyle as a highly important, controllable aspect of good health. Whether you are suffering from a medical condition or simply trying to improve the quality of your health, chances are you can feel better almost immediately by reducing your stress level. Learning to relax takes some time and effort, but the results of stress reduction benefit your cardiovascular system and your general sense of wellness. While most people need to work hard to accomplish goals on the job, learning to take personal time to unwind and reflect should also be a priority. One method of learning to relax is biofeedback, which has proven helpful to patients with headaches, sore muscles, asthma complications, and stress-related problems. Hypnosis can induce a deeper contact with one's emotional life, resulting in the exposure of buried fears and conflicts and relief from repressions buried deep within the psyche. Massage methods such as reflexology and Swedish massage work miracles for relaxing tight muscles and loosening stiff necks that have been caused by hunching over a keyboard or spending long hours behind a desk. You will read about these and many other relaxation techniques in the *Physicians' Guides to Healing*.

Once you have mastered the art of relaxation, you will find it easier to make some more positive lifestyle changes. For instance, there's no time like the present if you've been intending to quit smoking or get in shape. Take a long walk. Make time to play outdoors with your children. Choose fresh fruit for dessert instead of pie. Use the stairs instead of the elevator. Wake up a few minutes early each morning to do some simple stretching. Physical activity will do a world of good and will make it much easier to change other bad habits into good ones. The small decisions you are faced with every day can turn into a set of healthy choices. Some alternative practitioners advocate hypnosis to correct behavioral difficulties such as smoking, overeating, and insonmia. Living an active, happy lifestyle free of harmful habits is one of the integral components of good health and a sense of overall vigor and vitality.

Besides lifestyle, one major element of health maintenance centers on diet and nutrition: a great deal of metabolic balance and general health depends on what foods we choose to put into our bodies. Nutrition was an inexact science until quite recently in this century. Nobody, including physicians and researchers, knew for certain what our bodies needed to subsist and flourish. The discovery of the existence of vitamins in the late nineteenth century prompted the theory that our bodies need three main types of nutrients to survive: food that builds and repairs tissue, food that can be burned for energy (calories), and food that regulates essential bodily functions.

For obvious reasons, both allopathic and alternative practitioners stress the importance of good diet. Feeding our bodies the wrong foods can promote cardiovascular disease, digestive stress, and general malaise. The government has developed a set of guidelines for proper nourishment and categorized them according to four major food groups: meat, vegetable, fruit, and dairy. Until the 1980s, a "balanced diet" consisted of equal amounts of each of these food groups, with an almost equal emphasis on meats and dairy products. While traditional medicine was inadvertently preaching this high-cholesterol, high-fat diet to the American public, holistic practitioners were advocating and enjoying the well-kept secret of vegetarianism and macrobiotics. To holists, a balanced diet is one in which vegetables and grains prevail.

Nowadays the government guidelines for nutritional health have shifted away from the "four food group" grid in favor of a "food pyramid" in which the largest proportion of daily sustenance should be eaten from the grains category. The second largest category is fruits and vegetables. Then, smaller amounts of meat and poultry should be consumed, with the smallest daily servings in dairy and fats, oils, and sweets. There are more vegetarians—people who eat no red meat—and vegans—vegetarians who eat no animal products whatsoever, including eggs, cheese, and seafood—now than ever before; many people have discovered the benefits of eating low-fat and high-energy foods such as pasta, whole grains, and green leafy vegetables.

Another popular alternative approach to healing is chiropractic care, which is concerned with the relationship of the spinal column and the musculoskeletal structures of the body to the nervous system. The word "chiropractic" was derived from the Greek terms *cheir* (hand) and *praktikos* (practical). The main goal of chiropractic care is to help the body do its job. By correcting vertebral alignment, chiropractors minimize or eliminate interference to the normal flow of nerve energy throughout the body. This allows the body to repair its own systems and maintain good health without the use of drugs, surgery, or otherwise invasive medical procedures.

Chiropractic was conceived in an office building in Davenport, Iowa in 1895. Its founder, Daniel David Palmer, noticed a bump on the neck of a janitor who, seventeen years earlier, had become suddenly and completely deaf when he had bent under a stairwell to reach for some cleaning supplies and had heard a prominent "snap." That noise was the last thing the man had heard for almost two decades. That is, until Daniel David Palmer pressed carefully on the janitor's bump and immediately restored normal hearing to the deaf man. With one firm jolt, chiropractic treatment had been born.

Chiropractic health care is now performed by licensed practitioners in all fifty states. Common conditions treated by chiropractic include headaches, neck pain, bronchial asthma, stress, nervous disorders, gastrointestinal disorders, respiratory conditions, strains, arthritis, and migraine headaches. A chiropractic adjustment is a rapid, precise force (referred to as dynamic thrust) to a specific point on the vertebra. When applied properly, it removes nerve interference and induces the body to respond with an appropriate healing reaction. A chiropractic manipulation is a nonspecific procedure that resets bones, increases range of movement, and realigns joint structure. Some chiropractors also offer such services as acupressure, nutrition counseling, herbal care, and homeopathic treatments.

Members of the health care community have come to recognize that there is a place for alternative approaches such as chiropractic care, the alteration of nutritional choices, and reevaluation of lifestyles in our health-conscious society. Such alternative treatments as relaxation therapy, biofeedback, massage, nutritional and vitamin supplements, low-stress lifestyles, and hydrotherapy are now being prescribed by allopathic practitioners not only as preventive strategies, but as treatments for health disorders and conditions that already exist. For the active, overworked people of the 1990s, the wealth of new options available to patients and practitioners—thanks to the wider acceptance of homeopathy—have been embraced as welcome additions to the old, traditional set of choices. Consult your volumes in the *Physicians' Guides to Healing* series for a comprehensive introduction to the world of complementary medicine and for reliable, accurate answers to all your health-related questions.

THE PHYSICIANS' GUIDES TO HEALING

While homeopathy has been dismissed as "fringe" in the past and traditional medicine has prevailed, the past two decades have witnessed a movement back toward more natural and less invasive medical procedures. The benefits of both types of medicine are invaluable to complementary-medical practitioners who treat patients with every disorder—from strokes and hypertension to hernias and ulcers; from hemorrhoids and rheumatoid arthritis to sprained joints; from urinary tract infections to menopausal discomfort, myocardial infarction, and seasonal hay fever. Who decides if you should use traditional treatments or alternative therapies? Is it necessary to choose between the two contrasting approaches, or can you safely combine them? How do you let your physician know your preferences? Is it possible for you to work as a team with your physician to determine how your symptoms should be treated, how your pain should be managed, and how long-term health may be maintained? The answers to all these questions, and many more, are readily available in each volume of the *Physicians' Guides to Healing* series.

CHAPTER 1

Asthma, Allergies, and Food Sensitivities

*A wise man should consider that health is the greatest
of all human blessings, and learn how by his own
thought to derive benefit from his illnesses.*
—Hippocrates

The wise individual realizes that nothing in life is satisfying or even attainable without good health. You've reached for this book because you know this is true. You are interested in your health. The problems you've been having have forced you into taking action on behalf of one of your finest assets—your body. Because asthma, allergies, and food sensitivities are chronic conditions, you may have felt hopeless and very helpless at times. It is easy to become frustrated with the vague answers and contradictory statements that are often given about diagnosis and treatment. When we're in a healthy state it's hard enough to deal with such frustrations, but when our bodies are fighting chronic problems such as asthma and allergies it's even harder. We become stressed, frantic, hopeless, and sometimes give up. When the twelfth-century physician, Maimonides, was asked to treat the asthmatic son of Saladin, sultan of Egypt, he truthfully admitted, "I have no magic cure." There is no magic cure for asthma, allergies, or food sensitivities. However, relief and improved health are certainly in your future if you are open-minded and receptive to the variety of available treatments. Keep in mind the comforting thought that these conditions are all treatable, and that with proper and committed treatment you can lead a normal life.

ASTHMA

People with asthma have very sensitive tracheas (windpipes) that narrow when they come in contact with various factors. Their tracheas become inflamed and clogged, and the result is that they are literally gasping for breath. Asthma is characterized by an increased responsiveness of the trachea and bronchi (main airways) to stimuli (triggers). Common warning signs of asthma include shortness of breath, wheezing, chest tightness, a cough that gets worse at night or after exercise, rapid breathing, or a chronic cough. Other symptoms include dark circles under the eyes, difficulty sleeping, fatigue, a runny/stuffy nose, and headaches. More severe asthma symptoms that signal a need for immediate emergency care include bluish lips and drowsiness.

No one really knows exactly what causes asthma although most experts agree that heredity can be a factor. That does not necessarily mean that you will develop asthma if it runs in your family. What makes asthma all the more mysterious is that while some people experience only occasional bouts brought on by exposure to cold and enviromental triggers, others suffer from frequent attacks brought on by seemingly everything. In some cases, children appear to outgrow asthma as they get older, only to have it return years later when they are experiencing acute stress and anxiety. Still others, unfortunately, have to cope with chronic and lifelong bouts of asthma, along with occasional periods of hospitalization for acute episodes.

Regardless of the severity of a person's condition, developing a positive attitude can make a big difference because good health begins in your head, not in the drugstore! One of the better examples of how a positive attitude can make a difference is that of one of our most colorful and active presidents, Theodore Roosevelt. Roosevelt was asthmatic and sickly as a child and suffered from severe asthma throughout his life. Fortunately, his father encouraged the positive attitude that allowed Roosevelt to live not only a normal life but an extraordinary one. He religiously engaged in activities and exercise to increase his lung capacity and stamina, and never let his asthma stand in the way of his vigorous activities as a big-game hunter and president. His lungs may have been sensitive and frail, but he worked with what he had been given and managed to realize his maximum physical and mental powers. Talk about the mind/body connection!

Positive attitude? Negative attitude? Is your mental and emotional state really all that important or just some New Age mumbo jumbo? It is firmly believed in both the allopathic and alternative medical worlds that emotions do, indeed, play a role in asthma: strong emotions such as fright or anger can trigger an attack. Emotions may not cause asthma, but they can aggravate it along with other triggers that you will learn more about in the chapters on adult asthma and juvenile asthma.

ALLERGIES

You're sneezing and coughing, and your eyes are running like a leaky faucet. There is no doubt in your mind that allergies are affecting your life, but you're not quite sure how your life is affecting your allergies. What causes allergies? And why, oh, why, were you chosen to be the *sensitive* one? Allergies tend to run in families, and what you drew from your family gene pool (lucky you) is an increased vulnerability to developing this dysfunctional response. Because you were a "winner" in the allergy lottery, repeated and prolonged exposure to an allergen to which you are genetically vulnerable makes you, more likely than most, an ideal candidate for an allergic reaction to that substance. Say, for instance, that you come in contact with your neighbor's cat, and although you are sensitive to the cat's dander (skin, saliva, and dandruff), you have no immediate response except that maybe you begin to feel a little lethargic a few hours later. Because you have inherited the tendency to produce immunoglobin E (IgE, an antibody that your body uses to combat disease), these antibodies form in your blood and circulate throughout your system, sensitizing your system to the allergen (any substance that causes an allergic reaction).

Now let's say that you cross paths with your fluffy, feline friend once again. By now your immune system considers the dander from that adorable cat to be an invader, and your IgE antibodies gear up to attack it. The antibodies combine with the allergen (dander) to release histamines—a chemical in certain cells that, when overproduced by your body, creates allergy symptoms—into the bloodstream. The histamines then affect capillaries, mucous glands, and muscle tissue, making you feel entirely miserable. Depending on your body's ability to produce antibodies, this sensitization process can happen quickly, after a single exposure, or slowly and gradually, after many years of exposure. For the majority of people, an allergic reaction is a little like having someone tap you lightly on the shoulder and your responding by jumping out of your skin! Obviously your response would be viewed as exaggerated and inappropriate. This is also true of the body's response to an allergen.

In order to fully understand your body's skewed reaction, you must first understand that the body's immune system is set up to protect your body from harmful invaders. In the case of allergies, unfortunately, the body has gone overboard by protecting you from friends instead of enemies. When this happens, natural chemicals flood the body in order to attack the offending intruder. Your blood vessels dilate, your nerves stand on end and begin to itch, adrenaline and histamine flood the system: your body goes into a heightened state of alert. An intruder has been spotted on the premises, and your body is not going to rest until it defeats that intruder. Among the allergens that set off false alarms in your immune system are seemingly harmless substances such as pollen, dust, animal dander, cosmetics, molds, food, medication, and cleaning products. The list of potential offenders is infinite, but these tend to be the most common.

Allergens that are in our foods are called food allergens, or ingestants. Allergens that we inhale, such as dust and mold spores, are known as inhalants; and those that come in contact with our skin, such as detergents and cosmetics, are known as contactants. Some people mistakenly confuse irritants with allergens. Cigarettes and perfume are common irritants that provoke allergylike symptoms, leading some people to think that they suffer from an allergy when they do not. Although the irritant may provoke allergy symptoms such as sneezing, the substance does not stimulate the production of antibodies and release of histamines, so allergy treatments would be ineffective. Unlike irritants, allergies are rooted in the immune system and the effects extend to different areas of the body, including your skin, nose, throat, lungs, stomach, muscles, joints, the entire nervous system, and the brain. Some people even die from allergies. A severe allergic reaction, known as anaphylaxis, can cause choking, a drop in blood pressure, heart failure, even death.

Food Allergy

The very first person to record an allergic reaction to food was none other than the father of medicine, Hippocrates, who with his keen powers of observation noted that cheese caused an adverse reaction in certain individuals, although it provided harmless nourishment for the majority of people. In 1921 Carl Prausnitz and Heinz Kustner, two German scientists, made a major discovery about what causes allergies. After observing that Kustner broke out in red, itchy hives soon after eating fish, Kustner and Prausnitz decided to conduct an experiment. A small amount of blood serum was taken from Kustner and injected into Prausnitz's arm. The very next day, when fish extract was injected into the skin at the same spot, it caused an inflamed, itchy, bump to appear. When tested previously, the reaction had been negative.

The two scientists gave the name *reagin* to the unknown component in the blood that had caused the allergic reaction in Prausnitz. Based on this experiment, an allergy test known as the Prausnitz-Kustner, or passive transfer, test, was once used to diagnose allergies, although it was eventually replaced because of the risk of transferring viral infections such as hepatitis and AIDS. Not much progress occurred in the allergy field until the 1960s when Kimishige and Teruko Ishizaka, a husband-and-wife team of scientists working in the United States, made the discovery that reagin is a form of the antibody now recognized as IgE, which plays an important role in the allergic reaction.

Our progress in understanding allergies has come a long way since that landmark discovery, but there is still a long way to go. One of the problems is that health care providers do not always see eye-to-eye on the treatment and diagnosis of allergies. The most frustrating thing about allergies is that, unlike other medical conditions, not every test and treatment (except complete avoidance of the allergen) works for everyone. Most people must use trial and error to find the ideal treatment.

Why does it seem that lately everyone complains about having some sort of an allergy? Are you simply imagining it or do you just know a lot of people who seem to be allergic? You aren't imagining it. Allergies are on the rise in general, and, consequently, so are food allergies. Food allergies are exacerbated in modern times by the chemicals and preservatives in our foods, as well as by the additional stress placed on our immune systems by air pollution, antibiotics, hectic lifestyles, and the fact that many of us eat a very limited and repetitive diet that encourages the development of food allergies. In this book, the term *food allergy* refers to any adverse reaction to food in which the immune system is involved. If your nose runs and your skin breaks out after eating certain foods, or if you suffer from symptoms such as abdominal discomfort or depression that are linked with eating certain foods, there's a good chance that you may have a food allergy. However, it isn't easy to pinpoint which foods are causing an allergic reaction because some people may suffer delayed reactions to certain foods or may be allergic to more than one food. Because uncovering a food allergy is a difficult process, it requires a great deal of patience as well as teamwork between the patient and health care provider. However, the time and effort that you commit to uncovering the cause of food allergies is well worth it, because once the allergen is discovered, a treatment plan can be set into place that should produce unmistakable relief.

Skin Allergy

Skin allergy is a term that covers a range of conditions that generally fall into three main categories: eczema, contact dermatitis, and hives. Skin allergies can be quirky conditions, sometimes causing symptoms to show up out of the blue, last for a day or two, and then quickly disappear, while other symptoms may hang around to torment the victim with itching, swelling, and scaling for months at a time. Still other skin allergies come and go periodically for years.

Allergic reactions in skin are caused by a variety of factors, including exposure to chemicals, cosmetics, flowers, plants, and other substances. Skin allergies such as hives and eczema are often linked to food allergy and food sensitivity, as in the case of Marie, a classic example of how the digestive process is tied to allergies. Marie arrived at her health care provider's office suffering from eczema, muscle aches, and depression. Previous health care providers had told her that she suffered from various allergies and low blood sugar. Unfortunately, none of them had investigated her digestive process. If they had, the would have found, as her last health care provider finally did, that she was suffering from a yeast infection and what is known as a leaky gut syndrome (see chapter 6 for more details about the condition), which can generate an allergic reaction with symptoms such as eczema. A course of nutritional supplementation (with herbs, vitamins, and dietary change) was prescribed to correct her leaky gut and clear up the yeast infection, and she was completely free of symptoms within six months. Marie's ultimately happy ending is a perfect example of how essential thorough testing is in the treatment of any kind of allergy.

Allergic Rhinitis and Hay Fever

You sneeze . . . And sneeze . . . Sneeze again . . . And sneeze still more. . . . Take a tissue, relax, and read all about what's ailing you. Hay fever is a type of hypersensitivity to pollen, characterized by sneezing, a clogged nose, and itchy eyes, nose, and mouth. Hay fever symptoms tend to cause the most distress when pollen counts are highest—during the spring, summer, and autumn. Hay fever is often confused with allergic rhinitis (the official name for the majority of inhalant allergies), which tends to be more of a year-round allergy. Both of these conditions produce the same symptoms, although their courses are different. Hay fever is caused by pollen, while allergic rhinitis is caused by a variety of inhalants, such as mold, dust, fur, feathers, chalk, and other allergens.

Some people who are suffering from allergies such as allergic rhinitis or hay fever think that they are simply suffering from a cold. It's easy to get confused because the symptoms of colds and hay fever or allergic rhinitis are very similar. Colds and allergies can both produce nasal congestion, runny noses, and a cough. Generally, if the symptoms last longer than ten days and tend to have a seasonal pattern to them, you ought to suspect that an allergy such as hay fever or allergic rhinitis may be the cause.

FOOD SENSITIVITIES

What's in a word? While it may be true that a rose by any other name may smell just as sweet, in the case of food sensitivity versus food allergy, one word makes a tremendous difference.

In this book, the term food sensitivity will refer to any adverse reaction to food that does *not* involve immune system. The main distinction between food allergy and food sensitivity stems from the *causes* of the conditions. In cases of food sensitivity, the body lacks the enzymes needed to digest the offending food. It is simply unequipped to handle it. For example, people with lactose intolerance are often deficient in the intestinal enzyme lactase, which is needed to digest milk sugar (lactose). Because of this deficiency they will experience cramps, gas, nausea, and diarrhea after consuming milk products. Their body machinery is lacking the nuts and bolts needed to break down the milk sugar. It's the equivalent of feeding a coin machine with a ten-dollar bill. What does the machine do? It spits out the bill, of course, because otherwise it would gunk up the machinery and shut the machine down. And that's exactly what happens when you feed your body with food it isn't equipped to handle. Food sensitivity is a term that can be applied to all adverse reactions, including allergic, metabolic and pharmacological ones, to the ingestion of food. The important difference between food sensitivities and allergies is that food sensitivities involve the body's metabolism, and food allergies involve the body's immune system.

TREATMENTS FOR ASTHMA, ALLERGIES, AND FOOD SENSITIVITIES

An Overview

In the chapters that follow, you'll be presented with allopathic, or conventional, and alternative methods of treating specific conditions. Asthma problems are explained in great detail in the separate chapters on "Adult Asthma" and "Juvenile Asthma." While other medical conditions have been on the decline in this country, asthma, quite disturbingly, is on the rise. More and more people are seeking attention for this chronic, and potentially life-threatening, condition; and because it is a chronic condition, it often gives rise to feelings of helplessness. Don't give up! Help is on the way. The field of allopathic medicine has done important research to develop more effective medications with fewer side effects; research is constantly in progress to discover new and better products. Allopathic medicine is often necessary or extremely helpful in relieving the symptoms of asthma, and alternative therapies are a wonderful complement. Not only do some of the alternative therapies safely and effectively relieve nagging symptoms, such as wheezing and chronic coughing, but they support the body's immune system so that optimum healing can take place.

In addition to exploring the definitions of allopathic and alternative medicine, you will learn the importance of proper diagnosis and a precise course of treatment in treating certain conditions. All the details—what treatments were prescribed, what tests were given, and exactly how long it took before symptoms began to improve—are described vividly to give you the sense of being right there, sitting in the doctor's office, almost as if you were the patient. Let's take, for example, the case of John, an advertising executive who had been suffering from asthma for years. John had grown increasingly frustrated and dismayed as his symptoms, in spite of repeated visits to health care providers, had continued to worsen. Luckily, he had persisted in seeking treatment, and his health care provider was finally able to uncover the piece of the puzzle that helped everything fall into place. John had been suffering from allergies that had never been properly treated, and these allergies had been responsible for his worsening asthma. Having finally received the proper diagnosis and treatment, John's health improved dramatically. Seeing this kind of rapid recovery is almost as rewarding for the health care provider as it is for the patient.

In addition to chapter 2, which focuses on adult asthma,

chapter 3 gives special attention to the asthmatic child. The allopathic and alternative treatment programs that are outlined in the chapter on juvenile asthma will not simply duplicate the discussion of adult asthma. Although some treatments will be similar, many are tailored exclusively for the delicate systems of infants or children, which require special care. A variety of allopathic and alternative therapies can relieve the nagging symptoms that have been making your child irritable, cranky, and very unhappy. You will discover that alternative treatments are a fitting adjunct to allopathic treatment, but it is vital not to use them haphazardly. When you come to the discussions of herbal treatments and homeopathy, you will realize the importance of proper dosage, timing, and specific ingredients, and how they can make a difference. You will learn how to watch for signs that a treatment may not be working for your child so that you will know when to discontinue or adjust a treatment. This chapter can have a tremendous impact on your understanding and treatment of your child's general health as well. While you are learning about juvenile asthma, you may even pick up some tips about diet and nutrition that are useful to yourself and your children. Good health habits are for everyone, and this section is packed with diet and nutrition tips as well as priceless information about using herbs to clear congestion, balance the immune system, and cleanse the body.

In chapters 4 through 9, which are dedicated to the complex topic of allergies and food sensitivities, you will find details about the traditional treatment of allergies as well as techniques found at the cutting edge of science. Traditional allergists treat allergy as a condition stimulated by the overproduction of the antibody called IgE, and select tests and treatments based on that principle; they aim at the removal of suspected allergens and the treatment of symptoms. By contrast, the alternative practitioner views allergies as resulting from a variety of sources and bases treatments plans accordingly. Many alternative practitioners theorize that along with IgE-based allergy, specific non-IgE allergy also exists; an increasing number of allopathic health care providers also share this view, although this theory still has a distance to go before it is widely accepted. However, regardless of whether an alternative treatment or theory has been around for sixty years, five years, or is brand-new, it is important to consider that many people have successfully found relief from allergies by using both new and time-tested alternative methods when traditional treatment has failed to produce satisfactory results. This is not to say that traditional treatments don't work; it simply serves as a reminder that what works for some people may not work for others, and it is to your advantage to keep an open mind about treatment options.

Because the issue of allergies is so complex, this book examines specific allergies in distinct, easy-to-digest chapters. Special attention is given to allergies such as hay fever and allergic rhinitis, skin allergies and eczema, and food allergies. If you are indeed suffering from an allergy, it is important to pinpoint the precise type of allergy because each allergic condition should be treated in a specific way.

Many people think that they suffer from food allergies when in fact they have a condition known as food sensitivity. As we have mentioned, food allergy and food sensitivity are distinct medical conditions and are treated in different ways. After reading the separate chapters devoted to these conditions, you will have a much clearer picture of the differences and similarities. In these chapters on food sensitivity and food allergies, you will also find both traditional and alternative methods of treating symptoms. For example, if you are experiencing stomachaches and acid indigestion due to food sensitivities you could opt for many of the excellent and new nonprescription histamine-2 (H2) blocking agents that are now available, such as Tagamet HB and Pepcid AC. Both are excellent, relatively inexpensive, and effective products. However, they are not without side effects for some people. But if you are one of the people for whom these excellent gastric aids are simply not an option, you still have choices! Go directly to the section on alternative therapies and read up on time-tested remedies such as using slippery elm tablets to calm inflammation of the stomach or sipping a warm cup of ginger tea to remedy nausea and stomach upset.

Chapter 4, "Hay Fever and Allergic Rhinitis," provides a detailed discussion of treatments for allergic reaction to mold, dust, mites, pollen, and other common environmental allergens. In that chapter, not only will you find the most effective and recent allopathic remedies, but you will also find priceless natural remedies and countless tips on how to rev up your body's immune system to fight your allergies. You'll learn what trees, grasses, flowers, dust, molds, and mites to stay away from in order to keep your allergies in check. For instance, if you happen to suffer from hay fever, learn to love tulips because they won't make you sneeze. On the other hand, don't let your love bring you daisies and chrysanthemums, because they'll only make you wheeze. The good news is that you can sit under the pine, plum, and dogwood trees and you won't even sneeze once. It's so much more fun to learn about what you can do instead of to hear only about what you can't do, and you'll find lots of tips that will help you keep your allergies under control without taking the pleasure out of your life. For example, did you know that taking stinging nettle capsules for several weeks before the start of hay fever season can weaken, even entirely eliminate, hay fever symptoms? This is only one of countless tips that will almost make you forget that you suffer from hay fever.

If you think allergies are hard on adults, just try to imagine what it's like for an infant or young child. Allergy symptoms in infants can be much more acute than in adults, and immediate attention and treatment is always necessary. Because infants have such fragile systems and skin and because they are still growing and developing, their specific allergy problems are addressed in chapter 9, devoted exclusively to juvenile allergies. Allergies can interfere with growth and development and can even be life-threatening. Children also require specially regulated treatment programs, since many allergy remedies that work for adults cannot be used for children. Even natural remedies, as mild as they are, may have to be given in reduced dosages, and many should not be used at all.

If you suffer from skin allergies and eczema, you'll find much-needed relief in chapter 5, "Skin Allergies and Eczema." Many of the therapies are simple and easy enough to use at home. This chapter offers many treatments that you can prepare in your kitchen, and relief from symptoms is often as close as a short trek to the health-food store. If you suffer from the persistent itch of skin allergies, you'll find relief in the hydrotherapy section. Don't jump out of your skin! Just slip into a soothing bath spiked with aromatic essential oils or calming oatmeal or honey. You will also learn exactly what to put inside your body (in the form of nutritional and other supplements) to treat and prevent skin allergies and give you clear, healthy skin. You will also learn more about the primary role that the mind/body relation plays in determining the health of your skin. Beautiful clear skin is not cultivated from stress and tension. In fact, stress and tension can cause an increased vulnerability to hives and eczema. This is where you can benefit from massage techniques such as acupressure and reflexology, which offer relaxing, chemical-free, and safe techniques for soothing the stress and tension that can literally infiltrate the layers of your skin. Using their fingers like the most sophisticated tools, practitioners of these healing arts will restore balance and harmony to your body and, ultimately, beauty to your skin. By combining the best of both allopathic and alternative medicine, you may see tangible results sooner than you ever expected. And since you are attacking the roots of the problem as well as treating the symptoms, those results might even be permanent.

Welcome to the Industrial (and very toxic) Age! Industrial and environmental allergies are examined in detail in chapter 8. Chemicals are natural things, and all living things consist of chemicals. The danger occurs when we come in contact with chemicals that give us allergic reactions. Gases and fumes, smoke and combustion, solvents and other compounds can sometimes have disastrous effects. What happens when you become allergic to your workplace? to your home? to the world around you? The answer is simple, but not always pleasant to hear. Your body becomes a walking prison. And even though you haven't done anything wrong except to be in the wrong place at the wrong time, you are the prisoner. It isn't fair, but there it is. However, you can make changes that will relieve allergic symptoms. A change might be as major as leaving your job in order to avoid a toxic workplace, but most changes will be less dramatic. By learning about and using a combination of therapies—avoidance, protective clothing, herbal remedies, massage—you can assist in nurturing your body back to vibrant good health. You will also become involved in the process of choosing health—the many viable options for maintaining and restoring it—in a way you may never have experienced before.

CHAPTER 2

Adult Asthma

It takes your breath away. Your chest feels tight and con-stricted. You start to wheeze. Your throat clamps up and is desperately dry. You fight to exhale. You are an asthma sufferer.

Asthma is on the rise. Statistics vary, but general estimates indicate that from twelve to twenty million Americans are affected. People with asthma have very sensitive airways that narrow and become inflamed and clogged with mucus when they come in contact with substances that trigger an attack. It becomes hard to breathe during an asthma attack, and symptoms such as wheezing may develop in response to the narrowing of the airways. The degree of severity varies from one person to another, and symptoms can be mild—some people don't even realize they have asthma—to moderate or so severe as to be life threatening.

Enviromental pollution has been recognized as a factor behind the increasing number of people who develop asthma; it weakens the general health of the lungs, making them more susceptible to conditions like asthma. Stress and poor diet, common in these hectic times, weaken the immune system. Allergies, too, have been linked to asthma and can play a primary role in bringing on an attack. Even the tiny dust mite, a common resident in our pillows, mattresses, and rugs, must shoulder some of the blame; specifically an allergen in its droppings, which often acts as an asthma trigger, bringing on an attack. Unfortunately, dust mites have become much more prevalent in people's homes thanks to central heating and the lack of ventilation where there is heavy insulation. Most of us spend about eight hours a day in a bed thriving with millions of microscopic mites where we inhale their airborne dung and rest our heads on pillows that probably contain a fair number of living and dead mites and their droppings. The good new is that you can rid yourself of these pesky creatures or at least cut down on them.

At the present time, there is no cure for asthma. It is a chronic condition that can make us feel helpless, fearful, and confused. Breath is as essential to life as water. The fear of suddenly losing our breath creates anxiety and helplessness that interfere with our lives. It is important that you feel in control, assured that you will survive any crisis that develops from your condition. It may help to realize that millions of asthma sufferers are living active and vital lives. While this book doesn't promise miracle cures or magical potions, it provides information that will give you more control of both your asthma and your life.

WHAT HAPPENS DURING AN ASTHMA ATTACK?

Common signs and symptoms of asthma include wheezing, shortness of breath, chest tightness, a cough that gets worse at night or after exercise, rapid breathing, or a chronic cough. Other symptoms include dark circles under the eyes, difficulty sleeping, fatigue, a runny/stuffy nose, headaches, and drowsiness.

What happens during an asthma attack? During an attack

you feel as if your oxygen has been cut off and you are being suffocated. Depending on the severity of the attack, you may also experience feelings of panic and impending doom. There may be wheezing, coughing, or a whistling sound as the airways for breathing become narrower. The muscles surrounding the airways tighten like a coil, and the inner linings of the airways swell and push inward. In addition, the membranes that line the airways contribute to the attack by secreting burdensome, thick mucus that clogs the passages and leaves you gasping for air. It is the rush of air through these narrow airways that produces the distinct wheezing sound that is typical of asthma. Severe episodes must be treated as emergency since they can be life threatening.

Triggers of an Asthma Attack

In order to fully understand what asthma is, you must become familiar with some common terms. Hyperactiveness is an increase in the airways' responsiveness that usually sets the stage for an asthma attack. Obstruction occurs when the airways narrow during an attack. Triggers refer to the various factors that can set off an asthma attack. These triggers are described below.

Allergies   Asthma can be triggered by allergies, although not all asthmatic people are allergic and not all people with allergies have asthma. Many adults with asthma test positively for allergies. If you have asthma and suspect allergies, it is a good idea to be tested by a health care provider who is an allergy expert. For more information on allergy treatment and diagnosis, refer to chapters 4 through 10 in this book.

Food Additives   In general, people with asthma should avoid food additives. Asthmatics often have a severe reaction to such preservatives as metasulfites, which are common in factory-prepared foods, dried fruit, wines, and beers.

Sulfites can be found in any type of food, although their use is no longer allowed in salad bars. Another preservative called Tartrazine (FD&C Yellow No. 5) should also be avoided by people with asthma.

Exercise   Exercise frequently leads to asthma symptoms in some individuals. This is due to cooling or drying of the airways and the increased volume of air that is inhaled when you are exercising. It is important to note that this does not mean that asthmatics should give up exercise. Certain types of strenuous exercise such as running, bicycling, and aerobics seem to cause wheezing, while exercises that require short bursts of energy do not. Recommended activities include baseball, football, golfing, swimming, and gymnastics. Swimming in particular is an excellent exercise for asthmatics. The horizontal swimming position helps to move mucus from the bottom of the lung. An added benefit is the development of strong upper-body muscles.

Viral Respiratory-Tract Infection   Respiratory infections can damage the lining of the airways and increase airway reactivity, and asthmatics may experience increased attacks during this time. The best way to avoid this problem is to try to prevent colds and flu by frequent hand washing during the cold-and-flu season and by scheduling yearly flu vaccines.

Sinusitis   Many people with asthma also suffer from chronic sinusitis, also known as postnasal drip. This drainage from the nose and sinuses may increase the inflammation of already sensitive lower airways. It is a common asthma trigger, especially at night when mucus tends to accumulate in the lungs. A sinus infection can also worsen asthma, so it is best always to treat an infection with antibiotics if possible. Sinusitis may sometimes be linked to food allergies, such as to milk. If you suspect there is a connection, it is a good idea to get tested.

Stress and Emotion   Emotions can trigger asthma. Asthma is not caused by emotions, but symptoms can increase during times of stress and emotional arousal. Even positive emotions such as laughing may bring on an asthma attack.

Sensitivity to Aspirin   Aspirin can be a problem for asthmatics if they have nasal polyps. Nasal polyps are small nuggetlike protrusions of the membrane that may obstruct the nasal passage. Polyps are generally harmless, but if they cause discomfort, they can be removed surgically.

Environmental Irritants   Smoke, dust, sprays, air pollution, and strong odors can worsen or trigger an asthma attack, and you should try to avoid these irritants whenever possible.

Occupational Factors   Chemicals can act as sensitizers, bringing on allergic reactions in the airways. Once the airways become sensitized to a specific chemical, exposure to even the most minute amounts can worsen the asthma. Hundreds of chemicals have been shown to cause occupational asthma. Preventive measures include better ventilation and respiratory protection for people exposed to chemicals. Such measures are extremely important and should not be taken lightly, because once a person is sensitized to a chemical the only solution is complete avoidance.

Traditional Treatments   Allopathic health care providers generally focus their efforts on treating the symptoms of asthma. Because asthma is such a potentially life-threatening condition, it is essential for an asthmatic to be placed under the care of an allopathic doctor. A visit to an allopathic health care provider will generally include a detailed medical history, including patterns and intensity of symptoms, triggers, lifestyle, and a complete personal and family medical history. The good news is that health care providers have a lot to offer because allopathic medicine is continually researching new medications for asthma care. These medications are becoming more effective and have fewer side effects. What's more, allopathic medicine is the *only* form of medicine that should ever be considered during an acute and life-threatening asthma attack.

Diagnosis

Getting the proper diagnosis is the first step toward controlling asthma. When you first visit your health care provider, you will be given a thorough physical exam in which your doctor will perform such basic tasks as recording your weight, pulse, and blood pressure. He or she should listen very carefully to your chest, taking several minutes to listen closely and carefully. Depending on the health care provider and your situation, additional laboratory tests such as a urinalysis and blood sample may also be taken. An X ray of your lung will be taken to show whether there is damage or disease present. If asthma is suspected, you will be given additional tests. These might include:

Spirometry/Pulmonary Function Tests During these tests, you will be asked to breathe into a machine that measures your lungs' ability to breathe in and out. The measurement is then compared to what is considered normal for a person of your physical size, sex, and age group. These tests are also used to measure your response to medications.

Sputum Examination This test is used to check mucus from secretions in the lungs and nose in order to detect the presence of certain troublesome cells.

Methacholine/Histamine Challenge This inhalation challenge is the definitive test for asthma. Like any challenge test that has the ability to produce symptoms, it should be performed only under the close supervision of a specialist.

Exercise Challenge Tests During these, you will be asked work out on a treadmill, rowing machine, or exercise bicycle in order to demonstrate how your body responds to exercise. The results are also used to determine which medications are best for blocking adverse responses.

Arterial Gas Tests These are given to determine the levels of oxygen and carbon dioxide in the blood. The presence of too much or too little oxygen or carbon dioxide in the blood can signal breathing problems.

Sinus X Ray This is taken to see whether you have a postnasal drip or sinusitis problem that may trigger asthma.

Skin Testing If allergies are suspected, a skin test is usually given. During this evaluation, an allergen is applied either to the surface of the skin (scratch or prick test) or deeper into the skin (an intradermal test). In the scratch test, a drop of the allergen extract is applied; in the prick test, a drop of the allergen extract is applied and a small amount is pricked into the skin. In both cases, the area is observed to see if a local reaction occurs. You will have to remain in the testing area for at least a half hour in case the reaction is serious. For the majority of people, the area simply swells or a raised patch of skin (a welt or hive) occurs. If the reaction is more severe and the entire arm starts to swell, a shot of adrenaline will be needed. The intradermal skin test involves the injection of the allergen under the skin and is a lot more risky if you are very allergic to the substance being injected. It must be performed under close medical supervision in case a serious allergic reaction occurs. For more details about allergy testing, refer to chapters 4 to 10.

Monitoring Your Asthma: The Peak Flow Meter

Once you have been thoroughly tested and it is determined that you are indeed asthmatic, your health care provider will develop a total treatment plan for you. Allopathic treatment usually consists of evaluating the triggers of asthma attacks and working toward controlling, removing, or avoiding those triggers. In addition, medication is used to lessen inflammation and hyperactivity of the airways. Your physician will also introduce you to effective tools for monitoring your asthma, such as the instrument known as a *peak flow meter,* a small, easy-to-use device that measures the peak expiratory flow rate. In other words, you blow into the instrument and it measures the flow of air from your lungs. Keeping a daily record of your peak flow measurement, you can anticipate an asthma attack by observing when your peak flow values begin to drop. Your health care provider will let you know your "personal best" peak flow values and what steps you must take when they drop. To get the most from your peak flow readings, you should use the meter at least two times a day to see how your lungs are working and to help you recognize the signs of impending trouble.

In order to use the device properly you should be standing up while taking the reading. Set the scale to zero and breathe in deeply, closing your lips around the mouthpiece. Blow out hard and fast, while standing as straight as you can. Jot down the value you see on the scale. Take two more readings and record the highest of the three in your daily peak flow diary. You can purchase peak flow meters in medical supply stores or ask your doctor to recommend the best local supplier. By using tools such as a peak flow meter you can more fully control your asthma condition and feel confident that you are prepared to handle any situation that arises.

Preventative Measures

The ultimate goal of allopathic treatment is to prevent acute episodes of asthma, normalize breathing, and lessen hyperactivity of the airways. This goal is accomplished by taking the measures discussed below.

Evironmental Changes If, after testing and evaluation, your physician suspects that your asthma is triggered by allergies, you may be referred to an allergist, who will suggest, among other measures, making environmental changes. Upon a positive diagnosis of allergies, a plan of removing allergens will be devised and put into place. Lessening exposure to offending substances is the first priority. Air filtration systems, if carefully selected, can help some people lessen their exposure to allergens. Air-conditioning seems to help reduce the number of airborne allergens and allows you to control the household environment by keeping windows closed. Hay fever sufferers will notice that their symptoms disappear during seasons when pollen counts are low. If you are allergic to house dust, pets, or mold, taking such precautions as ventilating areas, frequently dusting and cleaning with adequate protection (face masks, special vacuums), and encasing mattresses and box springs in plastic covers to control dust mites will help. For additional precautions refer to the discussion of environmental changes in the chapter on juvenile asthma.

Medication Since environmental changes can't eliminate the problem entirely, medication is the firm foundation on

which all allopathic asthma treatment programs are based.
Most asthmatics benefit from preventive treatment with
medication that reduces inflammation of the airways. Medications fall into two major groups: anti-inflammatory and
bronchiodilators. Here are some commonly prescribed medications:

Corticosteroids (steroids)   Corticosteroids are the most effective anti-inflammatory drugs for the treatment of asthma.
They reduce and prevent inflammation in the airways and
decrease reactivity. Many people hear the word *steroids* and
immediately think of the dangerous drugs used by some athletes and bodybuilders. But these are not the same. The
steroids in corticosteroids are *not* the same steroids that
cause liver damage and sterility among bodybuilders. Corticosteroids are available in both inhaled and tablet form. One
of the benefits of the inhaled form is that it is deposited directly into the airways so that less is absorbed into the
bloodstream, resulting in fewer side effects.

Inhaled steroids   These include flunisolide and beclomethasone. An inhaled steroid is a preventive medication
and must be used regularly to be effective. Although it is
tempting to skip a dose or two when you start to feel better,
it is important to take your medication on a consistent
schedule. *Never skip doses.*

Oral steroids   These are beneficial in treating more severe
episodes of asthma because they are very effective in reducing airway inflammation and mucus production. They can
occasionally be used in short-term bursts or, in the case of
more severe asthma, as part of a routine treatment program.
The most commonly prescribed oral steroids are prednisone
and methylprednisone. Many asthmatics occasionally require a short-term course of treatment (two to seven days)
with oral steroids to prevent an emergency room visit or

hospitalization. It should be noted, however, that steroid tablets should not be the only treatment used to control asthma. They cause significant side effects, and ideally, they should not be prescribed for long-term use. Possible long-term side effects include:

- osteoporosis
- hypertension
- glaucoma/cataracts
- weight gain and fluid retention
- elevations in blood sugar (diabetes)
- weakened immune system
- growth interference in children
- muscle weakness or cramps, and joint pain
- easy bruising

Anti-Allergy Drugs   This is another group of anti-inflammatory medications including cromolyn and nedocromil. They are used to prevent asthma episodes but cease to work after an episode begins. Their use is best reserved as a preventive measure for those who suffer from mild to moderate asthma.

Bronchodilators   Adrenergic bronchodilators (beta-agonists) are medicines that relax the smooth muscles of the airways and open them up. They have very little effect on reducing inflammation, however. There are three groups of bronchodilators that are described below.

   Beta-agonists   Beta-agonist drugs keep getting better and better and are effective for a longer term. They are available in metered-dose inhalers (MDIs), tablets, and/or nebulizer solutions. Most beta-agonists begin working immediately and are best used on an as-needed basis for immediate relief of symptoms. Though the newer ones on the market have fewer side effects, some people will experience tremors, nervousness, rapid heartbeat, and increased systolic blood pressure. Be sure to inform your health care provider immediately if you experience any of these side effects. One of the newer longer-lasting beta-agonists, Salmeterol (Serevent) can last up to twelve hours, which makes it an ideal medication for those who suffer from nighttime symptoms.

Theophylline   Theophylline is another type of bronchodilator, available in liquid, capsule, or tablet form. Used to treat occasional episodes and as a preventive medicine, it is especially effective for people with nighttime asthma symptoms because it lasts much longer than the adrenergic bronchodilators. It is derived from the same chemical family as caffeine and has been used for treating asthma for over forty years. Theophylline must be carefully adjusted and monitored because too high a dose can result in such side effects as stomachaches, headaches, high blood pressure, and anxiety seizures. On the other hand, if the dose is too low, the drug will not be effective in controlling asthma. From time to time, your health care provider will need to take a simple blood test known as a theophylline level test to determine if the dosage you are taking is correct. Because food, medications, and other situations may affect the level of theophylline in your blood, this test must be repeated from time to time, even if your health care provider has adjusted the dosage at your last appointment.

Anticholinergics   Among the oldest forms of bronchodilator therapy for asthma, anticholinergics open the airways by blocking reflexes through nerves that control the bronchial muscles. One of their disadvantages is that they are slower acting than the beta-agonist medications, taking fifteen to twenty minutes to begin working. They are often prescribed in order to achieve longer-lasting effects after a patient has been taking an inhaled beta-agonist.

Immunotherapy (Allergy Injections) For those who can't control their allergic asthma symptoms with the usual environmental changes and medications, immunotherapy may prove helpful. Immunotherapy is a process of desensitization in which, as your doctor might put it, you are injected with steadily increasing amounts of what you are allergic to. Immunotherapy isn't for everyone, nor is it appropriate treatment for every form of allergic asthma. While some individuals with asthma may benefit from allergy shots, treating allergies such as eczema with immunotherapy is useless. You should also be aware that different allergists mix the ingredients contained in allergy shots in different ways. Some allergists may mix their extracts quite inefficiently, while others prepare theirs more carefully under controlled conditions that ensure potency and virtually guarantee that the allergen is free of extraneous material.

Immunotherapy does not work well with all allergies. It tends to work best for treating ragweed, venom, pollen, and certain kinds of dust mite allergies. Because each person's dust is composed of a unique blend of elements such as dead skin cells, mites, and other matter, some allergists claim that it's hard to mix a solution that will get good results. There is a tremendous variation in the samples of dust used by different allergists because they come from a wide range of sources such as vacuum cleaner bags and bedding. No shots are available to treat food allergies, and though shots for mold allergies sometimes work, they usually cause skin irritations. Allergy shots for animal dander are not advised since they are not generally effective and can even cause allergies to worsen or trigger infections; in such cases, total avoidance is the best treatment, with shots only recommended in the case of people who work closely with animals and therefore cannot solve their allergy problems by avoidance.

One disadvantage of immunotherapy is that you might be disappointed if you are the impatient type, because it is a slow process involving a series of injections given on a regular weekly or monthly schedule over a period of three to five years. If you are willing or desperate enough to take a chance and invest your time in immunotherapy you must weigh the disadvantages and advantages very carefully before proceeding.

During the office visit, you will be given a shot containing a very weak solution of the allergen and then asked to wait in the office for fifteen to thirty minutes to make sure that you don't suffer from a severe reaction. Before your office visit has ended, your arm will be thoroughly inspected to ascertain that you are not seriously allergic to the injection; if there are signs of a severe reaction, special emergency measures such as the administration of an injection of epinephrine will be taken. Otherwise, your initial shot will be followed by weekly or monthly injections of the allergen (in increasingly strong doses) into your arm. Eventually, a maximum dosage of one part allergen and one hundred parts solution is reached and maintained throughout the course of your treatment. If you suffer any discomfort after treatment or if you are taking beta-blockers, such as propranolol (Inderal) or nadolol (Corgard), be sure to let your doctor know. Taking certain medications while receiving immunotherapy can be dangerous, leading to difficulty in breathing, among other problems. Allergy shots should never be given during pregnancy, since an acute allergic reaction, including anaphylactic shock, can be fatal to a pregnant woman and even induce an abortion.

The typical immunotherapy patient is not likely to see an improvement for at least six months to one year after the start of immunotherapy, and there is no guarantee that the treatment will work at all. If no improvement is seen by the end of one to three years, it is advisable to discontinue treatment.

Sinus Care   Because asthma is aggravated by sinus infections and problems such as postnasal drip, it is important to treat any sinus problems. Treatment may include the use of antibiotics to resolve bacterial infections and the use of cromolyn nasal sprays to lessen irritation and inflammation. Ipratopium nasal spray can be used to reduce nasal discharge.

Performing a nasal wash is recommended for those with persistent nasal symptoms. One way to perform a nasal wash is to pour some saline (salt water) solution into the palm of your hand, then sniff the liquid through your nose, one nostril at a time. Then blow your nose lightly. To make a saline solution at home, mix half a teaspoon of salt in eight ounces of warm water with a pinch of baking soda. Place the solution in a glass or plastic bottle with a screw-on cap. You can also purchase saline solution in any pharmacy. Saline nasal mist solutions are also sold in pharmacies, and they are excellent for soothing nasal membranes, loosening mucus from the nose and sinuses, and restoring moisture to membranes inflamed by colds and overuse of nasal decongestants.

When it comes to finding the right allopathic treatment for your asthma, it is important to remember that it often requires a period of trial and error. Work closely with your health care provider to fine-tune your treatment program by discussing side effects and symptoms. You will know when a medication is right for you: you will feel better and experience a decrease in symptoms. Remember, though, that symptoms may come and go; you should not be lulled into thinking that you can give up your treatment program. With the right medication and regular care, you should be able to lead a normal, active life.

Alternative Treatments   Holistic medicine has progressed a great deal since the ancient Egyptians treated asthmatics by administering camel or crocodile dung. Yet contemporary alternative health care providers do not immediately dismiss seemingly improbable treatments—results are what count. Disease doesn't recognize boundaries, so why place limitations on treatment? While the allopathic health care provider will treat twelve patients with asthma in exactly the same way, the alternative health care provider will recognize that there may be twelve different causes. Because there are numerous causes, there are many ways to treat asthma.

Alternative medical systems recognize that a host of factors, including stress, environmental pollution, genetics, and diet, contribute to illness. Therefore, extensive medical, personal and lifestyle histories are taken into account when prescribing treatment. Treating the symptoms of an illness is simply not enough and accomplishes only half the job. In order to provide the best treatment, we must get to the root of the problem. This may involve a fair amount of detective work and a willingness to consider a wide range of therapies, but it is precisely these factors that make the alternative system of medicine a total, or holistic, approach to healing.

The alternative treatments described in this section provide various kinds of relief. Some therapies, such as herbal oil massage, may be very soothing. Others will invigorate you. Therapies such as diet and nutrition will attack the root of the problem and improve your general health. Not every therapy will work for you, but some will fit just right and produce positive results. Be patient. Undertaking a new therapy requires a period of adjustment—mental, physical, and emotional. The body requires time to revive and heal, so that even with the most effective treatment results may not be noticeable right away. Eventually, though, you should begin to feel relief from your symptoms.

Diet and Nutrition

The properly functioning immune system is one of our body's best friends, because it is there to defend you when the going gets rough. The immune system fights off and resists infection. In the asthmatic, however, the immune system often needs to be modulated; in the special case of the allergic asthmatic, the immune system, burdened by its reaction to food and other allergens, requires additional support to help keep it functioning property.

Holistic health care experts have witnessed the power of nutritional and other supplements in treating asthma. On the basis of the evidence, Jerry Hickey—pharmacist, associate professor at New York Chiropractic College, owner of Hickey Chemist, Ltd., and the former host of a television show called "Alternative Medicine"—recommends a diet free of fatty acids such as those found in margarine. It seems that these fats, when incorporated into the lining of the mast, or tissue, cell make the mast cell less stable and more prone to bursting, or what we call degranulation. When this happens to the mast cells, the lungs are more prone to inflammation.

Hickey suggests that his patients take a tablespoon of flaxseed oil (sold in health food stores) and eat salmon or other cold-water fish three or four times weekly; the combination of flaxseed oil and oils from the cold-water fish work specifically to prevent inflammation. At a daily dose of 1,200 mg Quercetin—a flavanoid like those responsible for much of the medicinal effect of foods and herbs—will further inhibit asthma by preventing the formation of leukotrienes, chemicals manufactured in our bodies that contribute to inflammation. In addition, Hickey recommends taking magnesium at a dose of 400 to 600 mg daily to relax the bronchi and ease breathing. A small amount of zinc (15 to 30 mgs a day) may also be taken daily, along with 100 mgs of vitamin B6 and 2,000 mcgs of vitamin B12.

Deglycyrrhinated licorice is an anti-inflammatory agent that also tends to be beneficial to asthmatics. You may want to consider adding green tea to your diet because it has a slight effect of dilating the bronchi as a result of its xanthine content; it also contains cathechin and gallic acid—two potent flavonoids that prevent asthmatic reactions.

In addition to following Jerry Hickey's diet and nutritional advice, you can make other dietary changes that help in controlling asthma. Here are a few suggestions:

- *Drink lots of water.* Water helps to keep mucus thin, so that the lungs can be clear and not clogged. You should try to consume at least eight glasses a day. Aim to drink a half cup of water at least every hour. Or bring along a large bottle of seltzer to work and drink it during the day until it is completely finished.
- *Eliminate milk and dairy products.* Adults (with the exception of pregnant women) should generally steer clear of dairy products. Dairy products stimulate mucus production and are common causes of allergy.

- *Eat moderately low-fat foods.* Eliminate sugar and keep protein intake to about twelve to fifteen percent of your diet.
- *Avoid caffeine, cold beverages, and alcohol.* Substitute healthful juices such as celery, papaya, spinach, and carrot blend, or simple lemon juice and water.

Herbal medicine

If you've ever seen a cat nibbling on plants to clean out its stomach, you've witnessed the power of "green medicine." Herbal medicine is the world's oldest healing tradition. The first record of herbal usage dates back over three thousand years. Long before today's chemical remedies were created in laboratories, "green medicine" was used to treat common ailments such as stomachaches, wounds, headaches, muscle sprains, and colds. The ancient Egyptians utilized herbs by smearing herbal mixtures on bricks, setting the bricks on fire and instructing the asthmatics to breathe in the herbal smoke. None of the herbal formulas we use today is quite that dramatic; however, they are equally effective for stimulating the body's immune system, increasing energy, normalizing body functions, and cleansing.

If you are going to use herbs for medicinal purposes, we suggest that you consult an experienced herbal practitioner. If you are working with a physician, always consult with him or her to be sure that the herbs are compatible with any allopathic medicines that you may be using. It is important to respect the power of herbs and to educate yourself on their use. If you suffer from allergies, be especially careful when using herbal preparations. If your skin breaks out in a rash when you use herbs internally or externally, immediately stop using that herb, or any herb in the same plant family. Never use herbs that are found in the wild, because accidents can happen when people misidentify herbs or use the wrong part of the plant. Always consult your primary health care provider before using any herb, particularly for pregnant women and children.

Keep in mind that herbs are composed of chemicals, as are drugs. Do not use herbs for a prolonged period of time, combine herbs on your own, or use any herb in large doses: even small doses of some herbs can be toxic. Never take a herb you are unfamiliar with or know little about. And always discuss adverse reactions or side effects with your doctor as soon as they occur. If you have any doubts about the safety or use of a herb, contact an organization such as the Herb Research Foundation for more information (see Appendix for address and phone).

Following is a list of specific herbs that are useful for treating asthma:

Siberian Ginseng Since ginseng is frequently used to normalize body functions and to restore balance, it is particularly recommended for asthmatics, whose immune systems often need to be modulated. Although ginseng has been known in the West since the days of Marco Polo, Siberian ginseng is a relative newcomer and has only been widely used only since the 1930s. It is a good herb for combating stress and supporting the immune system. You might take one or two grams of commercially prepared ginseng per day during times of stress. Do not take coffee, tea, soya beans, or turnips for at least three hours after using ginseng, because they tend to counteract its effects.

Although ginseng is generally safe for most people, it does tend to increase blood pressure and should not be used if your blood pressure is on the high side. Hemophiliacs, hypoglycemics, people with heart conditions, pregnant women, children, or the elderly should not take ginseng because of its tendency to prevent clotting, lower blood sugar, and raise testosterone.

Mullein　Mullein is reported to soothe the mucus membranes. It is an anti-inflammatory and an expectorant, a substance that promotes the discharge of mucus. You can rub mullein oil (five drops of mullein to one-half ounce of almond oil) on the chest to help clear congestion. Apply a hot towel or heating pad to speed absorption.

Fenugreek　Fenugreek is a complete medicine chest for lung ailments. It reportedly removes mucus, acts as an expectorant, and works to soothe sore throats and bronchitis. A cup of commercially prepared fenugreek tea may be sipped two to three times a day to clear up congestion. Pregnant women should avoid this herb.

Catnip　Catnip is not just for cats. Used as an antispasmodic it can be taken as a commercially prepared tea.

Sage　Sage is known to soothe the linings of the lungs. It is an expectorant, and it helps to eliminate mucus. It also has valuable anti-inflammatory qualities. You might take it as a commercially prepared tea. Recommended dosage:up to two cups a day for a short period of time. Sage is not recommended for long-term use. *Never* use sage when pregnant.

Passion Flower　An antispasmodic and nervine tonic, passion flower is especially helpful for those asthmatics who suffer from tension or nervous conditions, because it soothes the nerves. Take it as a commercially prepared tea.

Eucalyptus　Eucalyptus can be very helpful in relieving coughing and congestion. Dilute eucalyptus oil* with about six parts of almond oil and rub directly into your chest.

---

*The bulk eucalyptus oil found in health food stores should be used instead of the essential oil, which is highly concentrated and too strong for asthmatics to use.

Apply a warm compress or heating pad to speed absorption. Eucalyptus can be a bit strong for sensitive skin, so discontinue use if you break out in a rash. Before using the mixture, apply a small amount on your skin to test for a reaction.

Angelica Drinking one cup of commercially prepared angelica tea up to three times a day is said to clear congestion. Since this bitter herb tends to increase blood sugar, it should be avoided by diabetics. Don't drink more than three cups a day, and never use angelica when pregnant.

Acupuncture

Rooted in Oriental medicine, acupuncture is based on the principle that an electromagnetic life force, known as *chi*, flows through the body in a series of pathways known as "meridians." The meridians serve as conductors of energy, infusing organs and tissues with vital energy and the essential life force. In Oriental medicine, disease is viewed as the result of an imbalance or blockage of this nourishing energy. Chinese practitioners believe that the distribution of *chi* in the body must be altered in order to correct such an imbalance. During an acupuncture session, needles are inserted at a specific points along the meridians to stimulate or disperse the flow of *chi*. The needles are usually inserted about one-half inch to one inch apart. The insertion is relatively painless, although a slight pricking sensation may be felt. The length of time and style of insertion varies, partly because Korean, Japanese, and Chinese acupuncture techniques differ. Sometimes the needles are inserted and removed quickly, while in other instances the needles may be left in for as long as thirty minutes.

In a sense, acupuncturists are medical detectives, trained to observe body language, complexion, tone, and other clues that the body provides. The practitioner will check a patient's tongue to see if it is coated (in the case of asthma, it is usually coated with a white mosslike coating), and he or she will take the patient's pulse. This step is extremely important because, in Chinese medicine, 200 different types of pulse are recognized, and twenty-six of them indicate the approach of death. Acting as a keen observer and reporter, the practitioner will quiz you vigorously about your diet, exercise, lifestyle, and emotional patterns. After your initial diagnosis, a specific needle is placed at a specific part of the body, in an attempt to redirect energy and restore balance.

Acupuncturists view asthma as an imbalance of *chi*, the life force and energy that flows continually through our bodies like a river. To remain in optimum balance, *chi* must flow freely through the channels of our bodies, infusing energy into our organs. According to the Chinese, everything in nature must be balanced—hot and cold, dry and moist, dark and light, yin and yang. When are out of balance, we suffer.

The acupuncturist will work to restore the balance of *chi* in order to attack the root of asthma. In addition to placing specific needles along the meridians, the practitioner may also prescribe a treatment program consisting of patent Chinese remedies in which herbs are used to restore the bodily balance of yin—described as earthly and negative—and yang—described as spiritual and positive. The Chinese refer to herbs that are extremely yang in quality as "hot," while those that are extremely yin in quality are labeled "cold." Yang herbs such as ginger are used to treat "cold" yin conditions such as poor circulation and the flu. Cooling yin herbs, such as senna, are used to treat hot yang conditions. The practitioner will prescribe a patent yin or yang formula to correct any imbalance of these qualities within your system.

As part of the holistic approach, changes in diet, lifestyle, and exercise habits may also be discussed. It is important to note that acupuncture does not always complement other therapies and that other therapies you may be receiving can sometimes interfere with proper diagnosis by your acupuncturist because they change the body chemistry. Always inform your acupuncturist of other treatments you may be receiving, and let your allopathic doctor know about any alternative treatments as well.

How long does acupuncture take to work? Acupuncture treatment is likely to be required for a prolonged period of time, since the body requires time to heal; you should allow at least six to ten treatment sessions before deciding if you want to continue. Remember, too, that although there is no cure for asthma at the present time, this procedure might bring you pain relief, new energy, and milder and less frequent symptoms.

Psychotherapy

We are emotional and spiritual as well as physical beings. When the National Institutes of Health created an Office of Alternative Medicine, one of their first grants went for research on the impact of prayer on the recovery of drug abusers. You don't have to be religious in order to recognize that what we believe intellectually, spiritually, and emotionally can shape our physical health. Asthma can be aggravated by strong emotions and stress; and if we are under stress, counseling can help us to manage our stress reactions and resolve our problems more effectively. Asthma can be very frustrating to live with, and we may benefit from the support of a psychotherapist to resolve our feelings about being ill. We all need help from time to time, and there is nothing weak or shameful about asking for help.

Before you begin therapy, you should get to know the difference between the kinds of therapists and what they do. Just as there are medical health care providers who specialize in treating specific illnesses, so too are there different kinds of psychotherapists. The term *psychotherapist* refers to anyone who practices psychotherapy. A *psychiatrist* is a medical doctor (MD) who specializes in psychiatry. One of the main differences between them is that a psychiatrist can prescribe drugs to treat mental disorders and a psychotherapist cannot. A *psychoanalyst* is a psychiatrist or psychologist trained in psychoanalysis. A *clinical psychologist* holds a doctoral degree in psychology and has trained in psychotherapy. Clinical psychologists cannot prescribe medicine. They often specialize in specific therapies that may be helpful to people who suffer from asthma; these therapies include guided visualization, meditation and journalizing, body-centered psychotherapy, and family therapy. *Family therapy* may be particularly useful because the entire family is affected when one member is ill, upsetting relationships in the family unit. A family therapist can serve as a neutral observer and mediator, helping family members learn to support each other and to deal with the patient's situation in a beneficial way.

Support groups are another psychotherapy option that many people suffering from asthma find useful. Many hospitals offer such groups for people with a common illness. Sharing common experiences, problems, and useful information about an illness can make us feel better and less stressed. It is often easier to talk with people who share a common ground.

Osteopathy

Osteopathy offers a complete and thorough program with which to treat respiratory and breathing problems. On your initial visit to an osteopathic health care provider, you will receive a thorough evaluation, which is very likely to include X rays and blood tests. Environment, lifestyle, fitness level, and emotional and social factors will be carefully evaluated. In addition to the usual tests, osteopaths evaluate your posture and gait, and test your body for any restriction of movement. They also inspect your physique for skin changes, tenderness, reflex activity, and other telling factors. If they suspect that you have allergies in addition to your asthma, allergy tests will be given as well. Many osteopathic health care providers use the provocation/neutralization method to test for allergies. In this test, the health care provider places three drops of an allergenic extract under your tongue and then waits ten minutes for symptoms to appear. When the cause of the symptoms has been determined, a "neutralizing" dose, usually consisting of three drops in a diluted solution of the allergenic extract, is given. Osteopaths expect that the symptoms will disappear in the same sequence that they appeared.

After this thorough examination is completed, the health care provider will prescribe a multifaceted program of therapies that could include one or more of the following: nutritional changes, vitamin therapy, herbal remedies, homeopathic solutions, physical therapy, high-fiber diets, intestinal cleansing, manual manipulation to expel mucus, acupuncture, and hydrotherapy. As you can see, the array of treatments is vast; and since the treatment is tailored to the individual patient, each person will walk away with a distinct therapy program. While some osteopaths prescribe vitamins as part of an asthma treatment program, others don't believe that they offer any benefit. Because of these variations in therapy, it is impossible to predict exactly what kind of treatment program you will be offered when you visit an osteopathic health care provider.

Massage

Massage is a natural (i.e., nonchemical) method of stress management, a soothing manipulation of the body's soft tissues using a variety of strokes. If you suffer from asthma, chances are good that you've built up a great deal of tension in the chest area and around the arms. During an attack, the chest becomes tight and constricted. This tension does not simply go away after the attack; it builds up in your muscles and stays around long after the attack is over. Massage is useful because it helps to unknot tense muscles, stimulate circulation, and reduce the feelings of stress that aggravate asthma and bring on attacks.

Prior to a massage, you should be placed in a position to allow postural drainage—that is, your feet should be elevated on the massage table to a position where they are higher than your head. The entire back and chest area should be massaged with strokes that relax the tissues, muscles, and ligaments of the chest and shoulder area.

Homeopathy

Homeopathy is a holistic system of health care that recognizes the interdependence of mind and body. Homeopaths view symptoms as important defenses of the body, and they prepare specific remedies to relieve individual symptoms and promote systemic healing. When used in conjunction with allopathic medical treatment, homeopathy is a safe therapy for treating asthma.

On your first visit to a homeopathic practitioner, the homeopath will conduct an extensive interview lasting one to two hours. Follow-up visits will generally take around thirty minutes. During the initial interview the homeopath will try to find out what is unique about your particular asthma condition. For example, does your wheezing get worse when you're out by the lake in the summer or when you're in your stuffy apartment in the city? If you breathe more easily on a warm summer night than on a rainy winter morning, the homeopath will want to know this, too. You will be asked about your personal food preferences and your personality traits. Are you a sunny, warm person or are you cool and reserved? Do you prefer to sleep with your window open or closed? After a while, you may feel as if you are being interrogated. You are, but it's for the sake of your health, so answer the questions fully and truthfully. Rest assured that the information will be kept confidential.

The homeopathic practitioner needs all of this information in order to design a remedy exclusively for you. Homeopathic medicines are prepared from plants, herbs, and minerals, and may be used to loosen mucus, strengthen your lungs, and relieve stress. Dilutions, usually alcohol based, are shaken a number of times to increase their therapeutic effect. However, serious asthma symptoms, such as impaired breathing and wheezing, should be treated by an allopathic practitioner; and a physician should always be available in case of emergencies.

Homeopathic remedies are designed to enter the bloodstream directly through the mouth's mucous membranes. Since these remedies are fragile, your homeopathic practitioner will give you precise instructions on dosage, how to administer the formula, and even how to handle the medicine bottle. Dosage and treatment are tailored to each patient; and it is this individualized therapy that makes homeopathic care unique.

The following tips are useful to remember if you are taking remedies prepared by a homeopath:

- For maximum effectiveness, take one-half dropper of the remedy under your tongue and hold for thirty seconds before swallowing.
- Do not eat, drink, or smoke for ten minutes before or after taking the remedy.
- Avoid using mint (including mint toothpaste), camphor (found in lip balms), and garlic or onions.
- Do not use other medicinal herbal products at the same time because they will overpower homeopathy's stimulus.
- Keep your remedy away from direct sunlight, high temperatures, electromagnetic fields, and strong odors.
- Avoid using electric blankets when using a homeopathic remedy, since they can affect your body's electromagnetic field and interfere with the remedy's effect.
- Do not take your homeopathic remedy a couple of hours before going to the dentist, since Novocain may interfere with its effect.
- Always let your homeopathic practitioner, as well as your physician, know about any other medications, therapies, drugs, vitamins, or herbs you may be taking to make sure that there are no adverse interactions.

What should you look for in a homeopathic health care provider? First, be sure that the level of communication is good. The homeopath should listen to your concerns and explain fully how to administer each remedy. A good homeopath will keep complete and confidential records of your evaluations and treatments that can easily be transferred to another homeopath if necessary. Is the treatment working? Sometimes the first treatment that you receive will not work, and the homeopath may have to prepare another remedy. The homeopath also recognizes that some symptoms need to be treated by allopathic medicines provided by your physician.

Yoga

Yoga breathing exercises will strengthen and relax the muscles of the lungs. They can improve faulty breathing habits and distorted posture. In addition, yoga exercises can reduce nervous activity in the airways, which will result in less constriction during an asthma attack. By learning proper methods of breath control, less stress is placed on sensitive airways so that breathing in general will improve. Breath-control techniques can be learned and used anywhere or anytime to control stress, decrease the severity of an asthma attack, and control nervous tension. The meditation that is often part of many yoga programs helps to naturally alleviate stress and promote inner calm.

Because correct posture is an essential part of yoga, it is best to take a few classes before going ahead on your own. Once you have learned correct posture and breath control techniques, you can buy tapes, records, or books or design your own routine. Two particularly good yoga postures for asthma sufferers are the Mountain and the Complete Breath. The Mountain is an especially easy yoga exercise to fit into your daily activities. It strengthens the lungs, purifies the bloodstream and has a toning effect on the entire nervous system.

The Mountain Get into a cross-legged position. Raise both arms toward the ceiling in a prayerlike pose, with your hands clasped and your fingertips together. Keep your arms in that upward position while you breathe deeply and slowly for about ten counts. Exhale and lower your arms. Begin again. Do ten sets. This exercise can be performed in the morning before your day begins and again at night before going to bed, as well as at intervals throughout the day.

The Complete Breath This is a wonderful routine for those who are suffering from respiratory ailments such as asthma. It is reported to soothe the nerves and strengthen abdominal muscles. The Complete Breath fully expands the air sacs of the lungs, exposing the capillaries to maximum amounts of fresh oxygen. In order to properly perform the exercise, you must be dressed in loose clothing.

1. Place a mat or large soft towel on the floor. Lie down on it. Place your hands on your middle abdomen and rest your fingertips lightly on the navel. Breathing through the nose, inhale and expand the abdomen (fingertips should meet). Practice this Abdominal Breath slowly, approximately ten times.
2. Place your hands on your rib cage. Inhale, expanding only the diaphragm and the rib cage—not the belly. Contract and slowly exhale. Practice this Diaphragm Breath at least ten times.
3. Place your fingertips on your collarbones. Inhale only in the upper chest. The fingers will rise, indicating a shallow pattern of breathing. Now, raise the shoulders for more air. Exhale. Practice this Upper Breath ten times.

4. Place the hands, palms up, beside the body and combine all the breaths that you've been practicing together. Inhale, expanding the abdomen, the diaphragm and the chest in a slow, wavelike motion. Hold. Exhale in exactly the same order by contracting the abdomen, the diaphragm and the chest. Concentrate on what you are doing and pay attention to how it feels. Does the slow, deep, and satisfying breathing make you feel calm? It should. If not, keep practicing s-l-o-w-l-y.

Chiropractic

Chiropractic treatment is concerned with the relationship of the spinal colum and musculoskeletal structures of the body to the nervous system. It is often used to treat the stiffness and muscle tension in the thoracic area that are common among people with asthma. Loosening the thoracic area often yields positive results in the form of improved breathing and a reduction in the number of asthma attacks.

According to Isis Medina—a doctor of chiropractic (DC) who is associate director of the Gramercy Health Associates in New York City and adjunct professor at New York Chiropractic College, Postgraduate Division—"One of the fundamental theories in Chiropractic is that structure affects function. That is, as long as there is no interference in the integrity of the nerve supply, the physiology of the body is patent. Spinal adjustments relieve contractured conditions of the spinal musculature and overcome interference with spinal nerves." With regard to patients with bronchial asthma, Medina adds, "In patients with bronchial asthma it is quite common to find subluxations in the upper dorsal spine, specifically T1-T3. In those patients who have this as the cause of their symptoms, the disease will be relieved. Chiropractic is more involved than that, however. The doctor must identify where the insult to the body is coming from. Maybe it is an allergen causing the irritation, an inhalant, an ingestant, etc. One must find the cause of the disharmony to the homeostasis (the physiological regulatory process that maintains functions such as blood pressure and body temperature within normal range) of the body."

The main goal of chiropractic care is to help the body do its job. By correcting vertebral alignments, chiropractors minimize or eliminate interference to the normal supply of nerve energy throughout the body. This allows the body to repair its own systems and maintain good health.

Some chiropractors (although not all) offer additional services such as nutritional counseling and herbal treatments. Chiropractors must pass licensing examinations, and you should be sure that you are seeing a qualified professional.

TREATMENTS OF ADULT ASTHMA

Conventional	Alternative
Diet	*Diet and Nutritional Supplements*
Avoidance of food allergens	Cold-water fish three times weekly, flaxseed oil, magnesium, vitamin C, B6, B12, green tea, quercetin, deglycyrrhinated licorice
Environmental Changes	*Bodywork*
Avoidance of asthma triggers	Chiropractic, acupuncture, massage, osteopathic, yoga

Adult Asthma (*cont.*)

Conventional	Alternative
Medications	*Herbal Remedies*
Anti-inflammatory, bronchodilators	Herbs to relieve congestion and mucus
Sinus Care	*Homeopathy*
Antibiotics, nasal sprays, washes	Custom Remedies (Compounds of plants, herbs, and minerals)

Combined Treatments

There is a definite need for allopathic treatment when it comes to treating asthma. Asthma can be a life-threatening condition, and the best remedy for an acute asthma attack is always a visit to the emergency room for allopathic treatment. Alternative medicine is useful when used in combination with routine asthma treatment to help support the immune system and maintain the general health of the patient. Every individual has different needs. Someone who suffers from mild asthma will have different needs from the person who suffers more severe attacks. By combining alternative treatment with allopathic care, you may achieve a more individualized and balanced program of health care. A good example of how alternative medicine can be blended with allopathic care is a treatment plan that includes preventive allopathic medication to relieve current symptoms, monthly massage treatments to ease tension and congestion, and a yoga exercise program to ease the stress that can bring on an asthma attack; when congestion from a cold becomes a problem, herbal remedies such as eucalyptus or mullein oil applied directly to the chest are used to provide much-needed relief.

Here are some treatment options that, added to your program, will provide a comprehensive plan of both allopathic and alternative therapies. Remember that not all of these treatments will be appropriate or should be combined in every case, but they are good possibilities to consider and worth discussing with your health care provider. The following measures can be included in an overall plan.

- Use alternative techniques such as yoga breathing exercises to learn to breathe on your own instead of depending heavily on inhalers, which can become addictive.
- Design a medical plan that takes your mental health as seriously as it does your physical health. Use such stress-relieving therapies such as yoga, massage and counseling to help boost mental health and relieve stress.
- Use homeopathic remedies to ease minor symptoms. Homeopathic remedies do not interfere with prescription medications, so they are safe to use and can be a valuable addition to your allopathic treatment plan. Consult with a homeopathic practitioner to find remedies for symptoms that do not necessarily require allopathic medicines, especially for the sneezes and sniffles you may experience at the beginning of a cold.
- Learn more about herbs, and stock up on herbal teas that relax you, dissolve mucus, an soothe the respiratory area. Drink green tea to help ward off asthmatic reactions.
- Consider nutritional counseling to build health and vitality. In addition to removing food allergens and

preservatives from the diet, add supplements such as evening primrose oil capsules, which have been shown to be effective with asthma because of their antispasmodic effects. Take six to eight capsules daily.

- Double the effects of your anti-inflammatory medications by adding natural anti-inflammatory agents such as flaxseed oil, green tea, quercetin and other nutritional supplements to your diet.

- Make use of bodywork therapies such as acupuncture to remove blockages and help your body to heal. Your body can't reap the most benefit from the medication you are taking if you are experiencing stress, structural problems or blockage. Acupuncture can be covered by medical insurance if it is performed by a medical doctor or a chiropractor, and it often is. However, even if the treatment is not covered (because it is considered "alternative"), it might be worth the money if it helps you to live a healthier life. In the case of massage, many practitioners offer discounts when you enroll for a series of massages.

CHAPTER 3

Juvenile Asthma

Asthma is currently the most common chronic childhood disease for infants and children up to seventeen years of age, and there are unfortunately no indications that it will lose ground in the near future. Of the roughly twelve million or more Americans with asthma, the majority are children.[*] A child's difficulty with asthma changes with each stage of childhood. That is, an infant with asthma will have more difficulty than an older child because the infant's breathing passages are smaller. These tiny airways can easily become obstructed or clogged with mucus. But as the infant grows, the airways also grow larger, and symptoms may lessen as a result.

The basic defect that causes asthma does not go away over time; however, many children outgrow the allergies that trigger asthma, and they consequently experience few, if any, asthma attacks as they grow older. Sometimes it may even seem that the asthma has completely disappeared, especially among those who develop symptoms after the age of three.

Fortunately, most children do not experience long-term physical effects, but that does not mean that asthma should

---

[*]*Medical Tribune for The Family Health Care Provider,* 36, no.11 (8, June 1995).

ever be regarded without concern. Asthma that is not treated or controlled when the child is young can result in decreased growth and lung function, which will continue to trouble the child long after he or she has reached adulthood. Asthma can control your child's life or you can control it. As you read through this chapter, you will come across an extensive range of medicines that can help bring symptoms under control. The image some people have of an asthmatic child as sickly, pale, allergic, and withdrawn is, thankfully, a myth—and not a realistic version of how an asthmatic child actually does look and act. With proper medication and lifestyle support in the form of a healthy diet, a proper exercise program, and informed parental supervision, your child will be able to live a full and healthy life. The key to success is to start a sound treatment program and maintain it.

WHAT TRIGGERS AN ASTHMA ATTACK?

As with adult asthma, attacks are triggered by factors such as allergies, colds and sinusitis, environmental pollutants, emotional stress, even climate, and exercise.

Allergies

Many asthmatics also suffer from allergies. In allergic children and adults, the immune system is highly sensitive and will react to substances that are totally inoffensive to the normal person. Common substances such as pollens, house mites, dust, molds, spores, and dander from the family cat are sure to set off alarms. On contact with the allergen, the body goes into a state of emergency alert, producing chemicals that irritate the inflamed airways of the lungs and lead to symptoms. Many asthmatic children with allergies also suffer from hay fever or skin problems such as eczema.

Here are some questions to ask if you suspect that your child might be allergic:

- Is asthma worse in certain months? If so, are allergy symptoms such as sneezing, itching, or runny nose present?
- Do symptoms appear during visits to a house where there are feathered or furry pets?
- If there are pets at home, do symptoms improve when the child is away from the house?
- Do symptoms develop after exposure to a damp basement or room?
- Do symptoms appear when the carpets in a room are vacuumed?

To learn more about the symptoms of allergies and treatments, refer to chapters 4 through 9 in this book.

Food Allergies   Food allergies may trigger asthma, especially in children under five years of age. It is not always easy to pinpoint food allergies because symptoms can occur several hours after the food is eaten. It is a good idea to keep a journal, making sure to note the exact date and times that symptoms appear and certain food is eaten. If food allergies are suspected, take your child to a health care provider who specializes in treating allergies. For more detailed information, refer to chapter 6.

Exercise

Exercise can be a nightmare for the asthmatic child who is suffering from exercise-induced asthma. Children with asthma will tire easily and cannot exercise for as long a period of time as most of their friends. After spending some time on the playground or in gym class they may experience coughing or wheezing symptoms. This does not mean that asthmatic children should not be allowed to exercise, however. In fact, they are encouraged to exercise in order to maintain overall health and to strengthen the body. Good sports for children with asthma are swimming, bowling, tennis, and softball. Children also should be instructed on how to detect changes in their breathing patterns so that they will know when to take a break and then continue with the appropriate exercise.

Upper Respiratory Infections

Infections of the upper respiratory tract increase your child's chances of having an asthma attack. The best solution is to decrease the likelihood of respiratory infection by frequently washing hands during cold season and getting annual flu shots. Getting enough rest, eating a proper diet, and attending to early signs of a cold may also minimize cold symptoms.

Sinusitis

Sinusitis is a common asthma trigger. This infection of the sinuses can interfere with normal sinus drainage and cause increased nasal discharges, also known as postnasal drip. For sinus conditions caused by bacteria, an antibiotic may be required.

Gastroesophageal Reflux

Children who suffer from gastroesophageal reflux ofen have a backflow of stomach acid into the esophagus, which produces heartburn. The acid can trigger a reflex response that results in coughing or bronchospasms. Preventive measures include elevating the head of the bed, keeping the child from eating for several hours before bedtime, and providing medication to decrease or neutralize acid.

Emotions and Stress

People who believe that emotions cause asthma are mistaken, although emotions do indeed play a role in asthma. When your child is experiencing strong emotions, such as fear, stress, or anger, there may be a change in breathing patterns. Sensitive airways can be irritated by this change, and the result may be an asthma attack. Because of this connection between emotions and asthma symptoms, a child may quickly learn to suppress his or her emotions or become fearful of self-expression for fear of bringing on an asthma attack. Later in the chapter, we will discuss counseling as a means of helping your child to cope with this problem.

Environmental Factors

Smoke, strong odors, and air pollution can irritate the nose, throat, and airways, bringing on an asthma attack. Your child should avoid those irritants whenever possible. For example, secondhand smoke irritates the lungs, causing coughing and excess phlegm. It can cause children with asthma to suffer from longer and more severe attacks. Households with children who have asthma should be smoke-free. If this is impossible, then smoke only in certain areas away from the children's play and sleep areas. However, the best advice for parents is to STOP SMOKING!

Weather Conditions

There is no perfect climate for an asthmatic child. Some will experience wheezing on rainy, wet days, while others are more sensitive to a hot, dry climate. Some children are very sensitive to cold drafts and frigid air, and they should always have their nose and mouth covered when venturing out in such weather. For children who suffer from pollen allergies, the season when pollen counts are high will be quite trying.

THE INFANT WITH ASTHMA

An infant's lungs are tiny and fragile. A severe asthma attack in an infant, which can be triggered by colds or food allergy, can quickly escalate into lung failure. The infant's chest may get bigger and the face may turn pale or red during an asthma attack.

Here are some other signs to look for, which require emergency care:

- The breathing rate increases to over forty breaths per minute while the infant is sleeping. To calculate the breathing rate, count the number of breaths taken in fifteen seconds and multiply by four.
- Suckling or feeding suddenly stops.
- The skin between the infant's ribs is pulled tight.
- The infant's cry becomes softer and shorter.
- The nostrils flare or the infant makes grunting sounds.

During an asthma episode, do not give your infant large volumes of liquids to drink. Do not have your infant breathe warm, moist air such as the mist from a hot shower, and do not give your infant over-the-counter antihistamines and cold remedies. Always have an asthma emergency plan, which should include information about getting to the doctor's office or hospital, a list of people who will watch your house or other children while you're gone, and the fastest route to the hospital. Have available all of the information on your insurance or medical plan (identification, plan number) and on your baby's health, such as blood type and medications, for when you arrive at the hospital.

THE CHILD AT SCHOOL

Asthmatic children who are old enough to attend school face special problems. It is very important to communicate openly with school officials, such as physical education teachers, the school nurses and the principals. Provide your child with a written statement detailing his or her condition and clearly outlining any of your child's special needs, such as medication and taking short rests during gym class. Be sure to ask the school to notify the family—provide both parents' home and work phone numbers and addresses—if symptoms get worse or don't improve within fifteen to thirty minutes after medication has been taken.

The U.S. Department of Health and Human Services offers guidelines for determining whether or not your asthmatic child should stay home from school. Keep your child at home if he or she has the following symptoms:

- infection, sore throat, or swollen glands
- a fever above 100°F with a hot and flushed face
- severe coughing or wheezing that continues for an hour after the child has taken medication
- great difficulty in breathing; weak or fast breathing
- peak flow below sixty-five to seventy percent of your child's personal best, no response to treatment

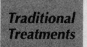

Traditional Treatments

Every treatment program for children with asthma must begin with a visit to a physician. Even if mild, asthma must be treated with medical care because it is a condition that can be fatal if it is either untreated or improperly treated. Traditional allopathic programs are effective in easing symptoms and preventing complications, and allopathic health care providers today strive to design a complete treatment program that takes into consideration the general health and lifestyle of the patient. The first phase of an asthma treatment program begins with a thorough physical exam that includes a detailed medical history, X rays of the chest and sinus areas, a complete blood count, and a spirometry/peak expiratory flow test. See chapter 2 for more information about asthma testing.

Peak Flow Meters

Because asthma is a chronic condition, both you and your health care provider will need to monitor your child's lung condition and symptoms. The peak flow meter is an easy-to-use instrument that can be held by a child. It measures the peak expiratory flow rate, which is the flow of air in a forced exhalation measured in liters per minute. Sometimes peak flows will decrease for hours or days before an asthma attack. By monitoring peak flows on a daily basis—on waking and before going to sleep, for instance—you can easily identify such a decrease and take precautions. Your doctor will determine your child's best peak flow range, or value, and what steps you should take when these values drop. For more detailed information about peak flow meters, refer to chapter 2 on adult asthma.

A number of medical specialists consider themselves competent to treat asthma. You may choose to take your child to a pediatric allergist (if you suspect allergies), pulmonologist (lung specialist), internist, or family practitioner as the primary health care provider to treat your child's asthma. Many parents prefer a pediatrician. Whatever type of health care provider you choose, it is important to discuss the particular individual's philosophy of asthma treatment. The doctor should have knowledge both of the medical issues and of your child and family. Is the health care provider available to discuss adjusting medication? How flexible is his or her schedule, and are appointments available on a moment's notice? If the doctor is not in the office, will a staff member be able to handle any questions or concerns? Is the health care provider willing to discuss combining allopathic and alternative treatments? Is the doctor supportive of you and your family? There is no time like the present to discuss these important questions concerning the health of your child.

Environmental Changes

If your primary health care provider suspects that your child's asthma is triggered by allergies (which is quite common), you should take your child to a doctor who specializes in treating allergies. The allergist will most likely administer a skin test. If your child is allergic to certain substances in the immediate environment, such as animal dander, house dust, mites, pollen, indoor pollution, or strong odors, you will have to alter the environment by taking the following measures:

- Use chemicals to kill dust mites.
- Replace feather pillows with ones made of polyester.
- Discard carpeting, since it is a magnet for dust.
- Use washable blankets instead of down comforters.
- Install a high-efficiency, particulate-arresting (HEPA) air filter.
- Reduce indoor humidity to less than 50%.
- Wash bedding weekly in temperatures of 130°.
- Use air-conditioning to reduce indoor humidity and control the environment.
- Keep clothes outside of the bedroom to avoid collecting dust.

- Clean furnace filters each autumn.
- Keep the family pet out of the child's bedroom and wash the pet weekly.
- Get your child a pet without fur or feathers. Think turtle or fish instead.
- Keep bedrooms, kitchens and basements well aired.

For more information about controlling allergies, refer to chapter 4 through 9 in this book.

Medications

Asthma medications are the foundation on which any sound asthma treatment program must be based. Finding the right asthma medication for your child may be a matter of trial and error. You can keep a diary to record how particular drugs affect your child's symptoms, behavior, and moods. Encourage your child to speak up about any discomfort or problems that occur when a medication has been prescribed. Special care must be taken to ensure that your child takes the medication properly and consistently, or it will not be as effective in reducing symptoms. As you will learn in this chapter, many of the medications have side effects. Some of them are minimal, but others are quite significant. Always discuss this issue with your health care provider, keeping in mind that your child depends on you for the safest and most effective care.

Here are some of the most commonly used asthma medications:

Inhaled Medications   The advantage of using an inhaled medication is that it delivers a drug directly into the airways, thus avoiding many side effects. Most bronchodilator, cromolyn, and steroid medicines are available in metered-dose inhalers (MDIs)—a hand-held, pressurized device that may release a medication as an aerosol spray. Most inhaled asthma medications are available in MDIs or "puffers," while others come as solutions for nebulizer treatments (see below). A young child may not be capable of manually operating the MDI well enough to deliver the appropriate dose of medication to his or her lungs. In that case, the child should use a nebulizer.

Nebulizer The National Jewish Center for Immunology and Respiratory Medicine recommends in *Your Child and Asthma* that children under four years of age use a nebulizer to administer most inhaled medications. A nebulizer treatment is given with an air-compressor machine. Pressurized room air is used to create a mist of the medicine solution, which your child inhales for approximately five to ten minutes. Cromolyn and most bronchodilator medications are available in nebulizer solutions. You can purchase or rent a small-volume nebulizer for use at home. Battery-operated portable compressors are also available.

Cromolyn A preventive treatment that must be taken on a regular basis in order to be effective, cromolyn seems to act by stabilizing cells that, on exposure to certain triggers, release inflammatory chemicals. It lessens symptoms triggered by exercise, frigid air, and allergies. Most people will not notice an improvement until cromolyn has been taken for at least four to eight weeks. It is available in inhaled form by metered-dose inhaler, nebulizer solution, or spin-inhaler. It is also available as a nasal spray for hay fever sufferers. Side effects are few, and include such minor discomforts as throat irritation and cough.

Corticosteroids (steroids) The most effective anti-inflammatory drugs available for treating asthma, corticosteroids help to reduce and prevent inflammation in the airways and to decrease airway hyperactivity. The steroids used in asthma treatment are not the same anabolic steroids used illegally by athletes or body builders, and you need not worry about the dangerous side effects of those anabolic steroids. However, you should be aware of significant side effects, which include growth suppression in children, a characteristic "moon" face, bone thinning, acne, and increases in blood pressure and blood sugar.

Corticosteroids are available in tablet and inhaled form. The inhaler is difficult for small children to use, and continued use can irritate the throat. A pacer is advised for young patients or those with coordination problems. It is a device that attaches to a metered-dose inhaler and holds the medicine while the child breathes in once or twice slowly. The pacer helps to prevent yeast infection in the mouth that can result from taking steroid medications, and ensures that young children take their medication properly.

Inhaled steroids   Inhaled steroids are used as a preventive medication, and like all preventative asthma medications, they must be used on a regular basis to be effective. There is little risk of steroid side effects, unless the child takes higher than the recommended doses. Possible side effects are hoarseness, coughing, and a yeast infection in the mouth called thrush. Steroid inhalers that are currently available include triamcinolone (Azmacort), flunisolide (AeroBid), and beclomethasone (Vanceril and Beclovent).

Oral steroids   Oral steroids are usually required to reduce airway inflammation and mucus production in more severe asthma cases. Oral steroids can be used in short-term bursts or as part of the routine treatment for those with severe asthma. Many asthmatics occasionally require a short-term—two to seven days—treatment with oral steroids to prevent an emergency-room visit or hospitalization. Some may have to take oral steroids for several weeks, gradually tapering off. But steroid tablets alone should not be used to treat asthma; they should be used only as part of a total treatment plan, if at all. It is best not to use them long-term because on such a basis they can produce quite serious side effects, including weight gain, fluid retention, osteoporosis, cataracts, high blood pressure, muscle weakness, stunted growth, and a weakened immune system.

Bronchodilators   One of the chief medications for relieving symptoms, a bronchodilator temporarily dilates, or expands, constricted airways by relaxing the smooth muscle and lessening sensitivity. They do not have much effect on inflammation. The three basic groups of bronchodilators are beta-agonists, theophylline, and anticholinergics.

Beta-agonists   Available in metered-dose inhalers, tablets, and/or nebulizer solution, beta-agonists are the most effective of all the bronchodilators. An advantage to using the inhaled form is that it works immediately. Possible side effects include tremor, a fast pounding heartbeat, nervousness, dizziness, and increased systolic blood pressure. Watch carefully for signs of overuse, because it indicates that your child's asthma is being poorly controlled: If your child is using an inhaler more often than every four hours during the day, or if the inhaler is used up in less than three weeks, the child's physician should be notified.

Theophylline   Theophylline is an oral medication (in tablet or syrup form) prescribed for a variety of breathing difficulties. It is effective for a longer period of time than the beta-agonist, making it a suitable medication for children who suffer from nighttime asthma symptoms. If your child is using this medication, your doctor will periodically perform a theophylline level test—a simple blood test to determine the level of theophylline in the blood. Many children experience side effects during the first few days of taking theophylline, but gradually they diminish or disappear. Side effects include irritability, restlessness, nausea, vomiting, a fast pounding heartbeat, headache, and difficulty sleeping. If these symptoms worsen or persist, or if your child has a fever from a cold or flu that is 100° or more, contact your health care provider. A prolonged fever (lasting longer than twenty-four hours) can increase the theophylline level and lead to more serious side effects and even seizures. It is important to find the lowest effective dose, since larger doses may lead to these side effects or even become toxic.

Not every theophylline medication can be used by children of all ages. There is no theophylline sustained-release preparation specifically approved by the FDA for children under six years old. Once-daily medications are not approved for children less than twelve years of age. For children under twelve who suffer from nocturnal asthma, a dose of twice-daily medication given at night may be adequate to control symptoms.

Anticholinergics Anticholinergics are approved only for the treatment of chronic bronchitis, but they have a bronchodilator effect in certain asthmatics. There is a very low incidence of side effects with anticholinergics, although cough and dry mouth are occasionally reported. They can be useful when taken after inhaling a beta-agonist to achieve a longer-lasting effect.

Immunotherapy (Allergy Injections)

Many asthmatic children suffer from allergies. If your child has tested positive for allergies to pollen, dust, mold, dander, or other inhalant allergies, elimination of the allergens is strongly advised. If avoidance of allergens and other options don't seem to work (and you've tried everything!), allergy injections might have to be considered.

Immunotherapy consists of a series of injections over a period of time—three to five years—of a solution containing an allergen to which the child is sensitive. The injections gradually desensitize the child to the allergen as the body acclimates, or immunizes, itself to increasing doses of the solution. Treatment begins with injections of a weak solution once or twice a week, gradually increasing in strength. When the strongest dosage is reached, the injections are given on monthly basis. Refer to chapter 2 for additional details about immunotherapy.

Sinus Care

Sinus care is an essential part of treatment for many asthmatics because sinus problems tend to aggravate asthma. Treating sinus inflammation and postnasal drip will result in a reduction of symptoms. Treatment can include antibiotics to combat bacterial infection, a nasal wash with saline solution or nasal spray, or a steroid nasal spray to lessen irritation and inflammation.

Emergency Care

It is important for you to act calmly and productively if your child is experiencing an acute asthma episode. If your child is having an acute episode, try to keep calm—doctors who work in emergency rooms learn to keep poker faces in the worst situations. If your nervousness is noticed, your child could experience extreme stress, which might further aggravate the attack. Immediately remove your child from the asthma trigger if you know what it is, and immediately call your family doctor or rush your child to the hospital.

Some things that you may think are helpful are in fact harmful, and they should be avoided in the case of an acute situation. Do not give your child a lot of water or any over-the-counter cold remedies without first calling your health care provider. Do not have your child inhale steam or warm moist air, since that will only add to the inflammation of the lung area. When you arrive at the hospital, your child may receive oxygen by nasal tubing or mask, repeated nebulizer treatments, simple breathing tests (peak flows or spirometry), fast-acting bronchodilators, intravenous solution, and/or steroid therapy. Hospitalization may be required, and follow-up treatments, which are likely to include extra medication, will often be necessary. To ensure that emergency help will be available should your child have an acute attack away from home, your child should always wear a Medic Alert bracelet engraved with critical information about his or her condition. Medic Alert's 24-hour hotline number (800-432-5378) will also provide details about your child's medical history to the doctor and other personnel who attend your child. For more information, write to Medic Alert, 2323 Colorado Avenue, Turlock, CA 95382 or call at (209) 668-3333.

Psychotherapy

Therapy is sometimes required to help a child cope with the difficulties of living with asthma. Taking your child to a child psychotherapist who is experienced in working with asthmatic children will enable your child to express concerns about the illness. Issues that might be addressed in therapy include any emotional factors that may influence the child's loss of breath, coping with the helplessness that results, building the child's self-image, and enhancing a sense of control over the illness and treatment. You might also want to consider selecting a family therapist, because sometimes family dynamics may contribute to the severity of the illness: when a family member suffers from asthma, the entire family unit is affected. Siblings of the chronically ill child might harbor resentment toward the ill child because of the extra attention, particularly during acute attacks and periods of hospitalization. On the other hand, siblings or parents may be overly protective, thereby insulating the child from life experiences that would enable him or her to develop into a healthy adult. Parents often suffer from feelings of guilt, anxiety, and fear, especially in response to the stress of asthma attacks. Sometimes parents may fail to discipline the child to compensate for the illness. The child may also use the asthma as an excuse for avoiding school or to manipulate the family into granting special privileges. The therapist can look at the situation from an unbiased viewpoint and help family members learn how to deal with a child's asthma in a productive and responsible manner.

In addition to considering therapy for the asthmatic child, mothers can benefit from attending parent support groups such as Mothers of Asthmatics, an organization that provides information for parents with children who suffer from asthma. Their address is: Mothers of Asthmatics, 3554 Chain Bridge Road, Suite 200, Fairfax, VA 22030-2709; for further information call (800) 878-4403.

Alternative Treatments

Alternative treatments for controlling or preventing asthma symptoms in children can be very effective, although they must be coordinated with primary medical care by a physician. Special care must also be taken to ensure that remedies are tailored exclusively to children's delicate and developing systems. Herbal treatments must be diluted, and some herbs cannot be used for children at all; bodywork therapies must be supervised by adults; and, in all cases, children should never undergo any treatments that they are not comfortable with. Encourage your children to talk about any alternative treatment that they may be receiving, and how they feel about it. If they are uncomfortable or experiencing any significant side effects, discontinue the treatment immediately. Always check with your primary health care provider before adding any alternative treatment to your children's program.

Herbal Treatments

Special attention must be given to children who are being treated with herbal therapy. Although most herbs are generally safe to use, it is advisable to work with a herbal practitioner who has experience in treating children, and you must check with your physician to confirm that treatment is safe. Standard adult doses must be diluted even when the herbs are meant for external use, since children have much more sensitive skin than adults, and high dosages can cause rashes and skin irritations. Herbs also interact with prescription medications and your herbal practitioner should be given a list of any allopathic and natural medication being used.

Homeopathy

The most common remedies for treating asthma are arsenicum album and pulsitilla. However, these remedies may not be right for your child. Although homeopathic remedies are available at the health food store, if you are considering homeopathy for your child, you should visit a homeopathic health care provider for an extensive evaluation. Homeopathy can be very effective in easing the symptoms of asthma, but it is not a substitute for medical treatment. Refer to the homeopathic section of the chapter on adult asthma for more detailed information on the use of homeopathy in treating asthma.

If you wish to purchase homeopathic remedies to treat minor coughs or congestion, here are some homeopathic pharmacies across the country:

- Hickey Chemist, Ltd., 888 Second Avenue, New York, NY 10017. Telephone (212) 223-6333; (800) 724-5566
- Ehrhart and Karl Inc., 17 Wabash Avenue, Chicago, IL. Telephone: (312) 332-1046
- Standard Homeopathic Pharmacy, 436 West 8th Street, Los Angeles, CA. Telephone: (213) 321-4284

Acupressure

Acupressure may be an effective therapy for children with asthma, since the acupressurist manipulates specific pressure points to release tension and improve breathing. An acupressure practitioner's fingers are used as powerful, precise, and natural healing tools to restore balance to the body. Like acupuncture, acupressure is based on the principle that the life force called *chi* flows through the entire body through a series of so-called meridians. Along these twelve major meridians are energy points that feed vital energy to related organs; beneficial effects are thought to result from releasing blocks of energy in the meridians.

There are four primary approaches to acupressure. *Jin Shin* was developed in Japan by Jiro Murai, who mapped a system of healing points based on his rediscovery of the ancient *chi* (also called *qui*) flow in his own body. In this approach to acupressure, varying combinations of acupressure points are held with the fingertips for a minute or so while the client is lying on his or her back. *Shiatsu* ("finger pressure") also hails from Japan. This popular method uses firm rhythmic pressure for three to ten seconds, and follows a sequence of points designed to unlock and energize the meridians. It is a very vigorous and energizing form of massage. *Zen shiatsu* utilizes points along the entire body, which are accessed by stretching, in order to awaken the healing channels within the body. Last, but certainly not least, is *barefoot shiatsu,* in which the practitioner presses his or her foot into the stress points to alleviate stress and tension.

In selecting an acupressure practitioner to massage your child, choose one that has experience in working on children. You will want to be involved in every session, assisting and observing, to be sure that your child is comfortable with every position and understands fully what is being done before or during the massage. Many of the breathing techniques and exercises that are incorporated in an acupressure session can be learned for use at home. Acupressure can benefit your child's breathing, and the sessions can be enjoyable, something to look forward to. However, if your child ever feels uncomfortable, the treatment will have to be adjusted and possibly discontinued.

TREATMENTS FOR JUVENILE ASTHMA

Conventional	Alternative
Medications	**Herbal Treatments**
Anti-inflammatory, bronchodilators	Custom recipes
Sinus Care	**Homeopathy**
Nasal wash, sprays, antibiotics	Custom remedies
Environmental Changes	**Acupressure**
Removal of asthma triggers	Manipulation of specific pressure points
Counseling	

Combination Treatments
An effective asthma treatment program begins in the pediatrician's office. From there, a plan can be developed that incorporates a variety of treatments that are tailored to the individual child. More and more health care providers are incorporating natural therapies into their treatment programs. By combining the "yang," or active, forces of allopathy and medical technology with the "yin," or passive, forces of nature's curative powers, we can balance the natural forces that contribute to good health. Emergency treatment must always involve allopathic treatment, but less severe symptoms can be eased by using a homeopathic or herbal remedy prescribed by an experienced practitioner. Counseling to resolve emotional issues and acupressure treatments to restore energy balance and improve breathing are two ways of accessing the health mind/body connection to restore good health. A really good treatment plan would include medica-

tions for controlling symptoms and inflammation, the removal of asthma triggers from the home, counseling for emotional support, and bodywork techniques such as acupressure to release the tension that a body under siege from asthma may feel.

Here are some of the measures that can be combined:

- Food allergens and preservatives should be eliminated from the diet; excess consumption of dairy products should also be eliminated, to cut down on mucus that clogs the lungs. Work with a nutritionist to design a diet that will eliminate foods such as wheat that may be related to production of excess mucus.
- Active children are healthier children! Sign up your child for a physician-approved exercise program consisting of activities such as swimming. Relying on medication alone to keep asthma in check is not enough. You should also concentrate on building your child's lung power through yoga, or use bodywork therapies such as acupressure to relieve the stress that brings on asthma symptoms.
- Use herbal treatments to clear congestion and fight off the signs of sniffles.
- Make use of homeopathic remedies to treat minor symptoms. Since these remedies don't interfere with prescription medication, they may be good complements to conventional medical treatment.
- Evening primrose oil has been shown to be effective with asthma because of its antispasmodic effects. Learn more about nutritional or herbal supplements that can help your child breathe. Food can be powerful medicine too!

- Learn about herbal teas and how they can be used to relieve inflammation and congestion. Consult an expert herbalist for recipes geared and designed specifically for children with asthma.
- Asthma is hard on parents, too. Consider signing up for a yoga class or stress reduction course where you can learn exercises to help relieve stress, as well as techniques for keeping calm in stressful situations brought on by your child's asthma attacks.

CHAPTER 4

Hay Fever and Allergic Rhinitis

Hay fever is what we call an allergic reaction to pollen. It is often used interchangeably, somewhat misleadingly, with the term *allergic rhinitis*, which is the official name for most inhalant allergies to substances such as fungus, mold, dust mites, or animal dander. What makes allergies like hay fever seem so complex is that some people suffer only seasonal reactions to pollen, while other people suffer a combination of seasonal reactions to pollen as well as perennial reactions to other allergens such as dust, dander, and even cockroaches! Hay fever is indeed a seasonal allergy, but those who suffer from allergic rhinitis have the condition during the entire year. What links hay fever and allergic rhinitis is that they are both inhaled allergies. Hay fever symptoms are relatively obvious: Most people really don't have to be hit over the head with a ragweed plant to realize that the watery eyes, runny nose, sneezing, coughing, sore throat, and ear pain and pressure that appear when the pollen is high are connected to their hay fever. People who suffer from allergic rhinitis may have to do more detective work to pinpoint the source of their allergies, although most have an allergy to pollen.

The pollens that cause the most alarm in hay fever sufferers are produced by weeds, trees, and grasses that are small, dry, and easily scattered. Ragweed is a major cause of suffering for people allergic to pollen. Other allergy-causing pollens include sagebrush, redroot pigweed, Russian thistle, and English plaintain. Grass, too, produces allergic pollen; and it is best to stay away from Kentucky bluegrass, redtop, orchard, and sweet vernon if you are pollen-sensitive. Oak and ash trees produce high levels of allergic pollen, and so do maple, elm, hickory, and pecan. These trees look pretty, but it may be better to stay far away from them if you want to breathe easily.

If you suffer from allergic rhinitis, you may be allergic to a member of the fungi family known as mold, which may cause allergic rhinitis when the mold spores are inhaled. Molds tend to thrive in places where there is a lot of moisture and oxygen, for instance under rotting logs and fallen leaves. They grow on house plants, and in damp basements, closets, and musty bathrooms. They can also be found in humidifiers and air conditioners that are not cleaned thoroughly and often. Molds tend to be a year-round allergy, especially in areas of the country that stay warm throughout the year, since unlike pollen they won't disappear after the first hint of cold weather. Some molds can even survive at below-freezing temperatures. Avoid foods that contain fungi or yeast, such as cheese, mushrooms, soy sauce, beer, fruit juices, pickles, tofu, vinegar, tomato products, and dried fruits, since these foods can cause an allergic reaction in individuals sensitive to mold. If you suspect that a food in your refrigerator is spoiled, don't smell it; simply throw it out. Inhaling the spores could set off your allergies. Try to shop often to ensure that your foods are fresh, since food that sits in your kitchen is vulnerable to mold. Speaking of vulnerability, don't eat a heavy-sugar diet because molds thrive on sugar inside and outside your body.

By far the most common cause of year-round allergic rhinitis is house dust. This is a particularly frustrating allergy, because it is impossible to escape even in the cleanest of houses; and even in the most minute amounts, dust can cause an allergic reaction. House dust also includes dust mites— microscopic insects—that thrive in our carpets, mattresses, and furniture. These mites and their waste products are major irritants. If you are sleeping on a pillow filled with dust mites and their waste, you are sure to have a hard time avoiding allergies. (Helpful hint: Buy polyester pillows instead of down.)

Another major source of allergic rhinitis could be your dog or cat. It's not the luxurious coat that they are wearing that is making you sneeze; it's the dander from the saliva that they deposit on their coats while cleaning themselves. Cats are the worst offenders, because they are meticulous creatures that preen often and quite well. The more an animal cleans itself, the more you sneeze. Sprays exist that can be applied directly to animal fur and reduce the harmful dander. Before using, consult your pet's veterinarian as well as your physician.

Traditional Treatments   If you suspect that you are suffering from hay fever or allergic rhinitis, you should visit your health care provider for testing. Before your first visit, ask the receptionist for an estimate of how long this will take. Most initial visits for allergy testing last as long as two hours or more, so don't make an appointment for a day when you will be rushed. Come prepared with related medical records, answers about your family history of allergy, notes about your symptoms, and details about any previous treatments you may have been given for allergies of any kind.

Diagnosing Your Allergy

During your initial visit, your health care provider will take a thorough personal and family medical history. Since much of the diagnosis depends on the doctor's access to an accurate record, as well as on a complete discussion of symptoms, be sure that you are doing your share by offering every bit of information that is available. Start by telling your doctor what symptoms were causing you enough concern to make an appointmnent. Are you in pain? Does your nose run? When and where does it run? Try to remember exactly when your symptoms began. Tell your health care provider if the problem comes and goes or is constant. Does it interfere with your work? Is it food related? Cover all bases and try not to leave anything out, no matter how minor it seems to you. Once your health care provider has a complete medical and personal history, a thorough physical examination will be conducted, to search your body for clues. Your head, ears, eyes, nose, throat, neck, lungs, heart, abdomen, and skin will be examined for signs of allergy or other possible causes of your symptoms.

In addition to the physical exam, several tests may be given to determine the cause of allergies.

Prick Test   Prick tests are the safest skin tests because, even if you are extremely allergic, they are very unlikely to provoke a serious reaction. In this test, a drop of solution from each allergen—up to thirty-five possible allergens can be tested at once—is applied to the skin, which is pricked with a needlelike object. Reactions are noted and recorded. If you are sensitive to the allergen, slight swelling and itching will occur almost immediately. For some people, a different sort of reaction known as a late-phase reaction can set in, producing a large, painful lump. Late-phase reactions are important to note because they are a major factor in the development of chronic allergic conditions in which the patient never seems to be completely free of symptoms. In such cases, a person has an acute reaction to an allergen on immediate contact and then recovers—only to have another reaction to the substance between four and twelve hours after exposure as a result of a later release of chemicals from the mast cells. Although late-phase reactions can make it harder to pinpoint the cause of an allergy, medications can be prescribed to block those reactions once their cause is understood.

Nasal Smear   In this test, a person blows his or her nose onto a plastic sheet, so that the sample can be examined for high numbers of white blood cells that are usually present with an allergy. Your health care provider should also examine the physical structure of your nose to see if the mucous membranes are swollen or discolored, as is often the case in allergy sufferers.

Scratch Test   This test is conducted in a manner similar to the prick test. A small scratch is made on the skin of the arm with a very fine needle. A drop of solution is placed on it and reactions are noted.

Intradermal   This test is usually given if you do not react to the prick test. A testing solution is injected under your skin rather than being placed on top of it. Due to the risk of a life-threatening allergic reaction to the testing solution, this test is never given when the prick test is positive. Intradermals are often used when a doctor suspects that a sensitivity is present in spite of negative results from a scratch or prick test.

Blood Tests Blood tests for allergies use a blood sample to determine the amount of specific IgE antibodies in the blood. These tests are expensive and not as sensitive as skin testing.

The Three Basic Therapies

The three basic traditional methods of treating allergies are avoidance, immunotherapy, and medications.

Avoidance Avoiding the allergen is the number one method because it eliminates the trigger entirely and therefore curbs your symptoms. If your test indicates that you have hay fever, you might want to take special precautions, such as wearing glasses or sunglasses outdoors to protect your eyes from pollen, and staying indoors between 5 A.M. and 10 A.M. when pollen levels are at their highest. You can also try rubbing a dab of vitamin E oil on your nostrils to make it harder for the pollen to penetrate your nose. During pollen season, try to wash your hands every time you come in from outdoors, and bathe before going to bed so that you don't take the pollen into bed with you. If you're thinking of moving to escape from pollen, forget about it. There are no areas of the country that can claim to be entirely allergy-free. Instead of moving, you might want to take vacations when the pollen count in your area is highest. If you're allergic to other inhalants, such as mold and dust, complete removal of allergens can be impossible; but there are measures that you can take to cut down on exposure to those substances. Refer to chapter 2 on environmental changes for more details on how to cope with inhaled allergens.

Immunotherapy Allergy injections are a possibility when you find that you can't avoid your allergens. This form of treatment is used to treat hay fever and allergic rhinitis when other measures have failed. As explained in chapter 1 of this book, immunization is a process of desensitization in which you are injected with increasingly larger doses of substances to which you are allergic. It works best for pollen, ragweed, and dust mite allergies. Refer to the immunotherapy section of chapter 1 for more details.

Medications   Medications are used to relieve symptoms and make patients more comfortable during their daily activities. People who suffer from severe symptoms would find it hard to function if it were not for medications that clear their stuffy noses and heads and relieve teary eyes.

Although they do not address the underlying cause of the allergy, antihistamines, decongestants, and prescription nasal sprays can reduce such symptoms as watery eyes, runny nose, and congestion. Common antihistamines used to treat hay fever and allergy symptoms are brompheniramine, chlorpheniramine, diphenhydramine, and phenyltoloxamine. A prescription antihistamine by the name of Seldane (terfenadine) was one of the first antihistamines that did not cause drowsiness. Another antihistamine available by prescription that does not have sedating qualities is Hismanal (astemizole). The downside of these two antihistamines is that they can have very serious side effects if used in higher dosages than advised by the manufacturer, or if used by patients with significant liver problems or those who take the drugs ketoconazole and erythromycin. For these reasons and other side effects such as dry nose, mouth, and throat, some people might prefer to put up with the drowsiness produced by over-the-counter medications.

Decongestants are helpful for shrinking swollen nasal passages, but they are not without side effects. Regular use can cause irritability, headaches, and dizziness, and they can become quite addictive: Once you stop taking them, your nose may feel stuffy again and you may have to start using them again. This can quickly evolve into a vicious cycle leading to dependence on decongestants in order to breathe more easily. Most over-the-counter (OTC) allergy drugs, including some familiar brand names such as Allerest, Actifed, Tavist-D and Benadryl 25, contain both an antihistamine and a decongestant. Whenever you take any medication, whether nonprescription or prescription, always read the instructions carefully, especially for exact dosage, drug interaction precautions, the time required for the medication to become effective after ingestion, and expiration dates. If you want to know more about side effects, risks, and interactions consult a reference book on medications such as *The Complete Drug Reference,* which is available from Consumer Reports, Box 10637, Des Moines, IA 50336; or call (515) 237-4903 for further information. Drug reference guides can also be found at your local library.

Alternative Treatments

If, after having taken proper measures to avoid your allergens, you don't relish the idea of relying only on standard pharmaceuticals to control your allergies, you might want to try alternative therapies. In this chapter you will learn how natural foods can be used as a defense against the daily assault of irritating allergens. A detailed presentation of herbal treatments suggests ways to use herbs to relieve nasal and sinus congestion and watery eyes. Acupuncture, meditation, and homeopathy are also discussed as potential allies in the battle to restore your body's equilibrium. Although it is not likely that you'll want—or even need—to use all of the therapies discussed here, you will soon learn that making even a few changes in your therapy or daily routine may yield beneficial results.

Acupuncture

During your initial office visit, the acupuncturist will observe and examine you very carefully. Working with a holistic understanding of how body (including specific organs), mind, and emotions are interrelated, the practitioner examines the body closely for clues about which organs or underlying systems may be malfunctioning as a result of a blocked flow of energy through the body.

- Different pulses in the body compare to different organs. The practitioner checks pulses at three different places on the arm, using different degrees of pressure in search of energy blockages in corresponding organs.
- The condition of the tongue provides clues about general and more specific health problems. The practitioner carefully observes its color and whether it is coated.
- Allergic reactions are shown in skin eruptions or irritation such as hives, eczema, and contact dermatitis. The practitioner will check the face for skin tone and color that indicate allergies as well as underlying systemic problems.
- Illness, allergies, and other factors influence how we smell. The practitioner will check specific body odors that may indicate a fever or other disorders.
- The tone of voice we use can be a clue to our emotional state. The practitioner is highly trained to detect the most subtle nuances.

Your answers to the practitioner's questions will reveal a great deal about what may be causing your symptoms. Where you work, how much energy you have at certain times of the day, and what temperatures you are most comfortable with: all these provide clues as to individual patterns that can lead to imbalance. The main factor in allergies, in terms of Chinese medicine, is the condition of the patient's normal *chi,* or life force. If the *chi* is unbalanced, coping with the external world becomes extremely difficult. After assessing your particular situation, the acupuncturist will devise a specific plan for you. In addition to working to unblock energy with needles inserted in the meridians (the channels in the body through which life flows), the acupuncturist may prescribe changes in diet and lifestyle. You may see results very quickly, but on the other hand your improvement may be slow and gradual. The course of allergies is not easy to predict, and some allergies can be treated more easily than others. With each session, the practitioner will diagnose and adjust treatments until the body's energy flow is in balance and health is restored.

Herbal Treatments

Herbs can be a great help in relieving allergies in conjunction with allopathic medicine. They can be used to unblock clogged nasal passages, clear chest congestion, and strengthen the immune system.

The next time you are experiencing a runny nose and watery eyes, you might want to stop at a reputable health-food store. Herbalists believe that the human body is its own best health care provider, and that they can assist nature in healing through the proper use of herbal remedies. Since many allergies such as hay fever spring from natural substances— pollen, for example—why not let nature take its course and use a natural remedy to heal? Many store owners are very knowledgeable about herbal teas and remedies, and they can give you valuable pointers about dosage and various combined treatments. Most health-food stores stock ready-made allergy formulas, although it may take trial and error to find the right remedy for you. But you must be careful to monitor use for any negative side effects.

The following herbs are often used to treat hay fever and allergic rhinitis. Most remedies are safe for most people—although children, pregnant women, and those with special medical conditions should always check with their doctors before using herbal preparations. Your physician can help ensure that a particular remedy is appropriate for your condition.

Stinging Nettle Stinging nettle is the champion of herbs for treating hay fever symptoms. As a preventive measure taken two or three weeks before hay-fever season begins, freeze-dried stinging nettle capsules can lessen symptoms or even prevent full-blown allergy symptoms from occurring. Stinging nettle capsules are readily available in most health food stores. Usage recommendation: Take one or two 300 mg. capsules daily of freeze-dried leaves to stop or prevent allergy symptoms during hay fever season, upon the approval of your healthcare provider. Note: Nettle has a slightly diuretic effect. Do not, however, give this herb to children, the elderly, or pregnant women.

Angelica Angelica has long been used by Chinese herbalists in the treatment of hay fever, eczema, and allergies connected to dust, dander, pollens, and other substances. It inhibits the production of allergic antibodies (IgE), which are usually elevated more significantly among allergic individuals than among people without allergies. Angelica can be taken as a commercially prepared tea for symptom relief, but do not consume more than three cups per day. Elderly people, pregnant women, and children should not take it.

Elder Elder is quite common in the countryside, and its leaves, stems and flowers are used in various herbal treatments, although for safety's sake, only commercially prepared elder should be used for herbal treatments. Elder flowers are an excellent remedy for a variety of respiratory conditions since it helps to ease congestion and inflammation. The berries are an also an excellent source of vitamin C.

Ginkgo Extracted from the leaves and nuts of the ginkgo tree, ginkgo is an antioxidant and expectorant that expels mucus from the lungs. Ginkgo must be used with great care since it can be toxic. Consult a herbalist for guidelines.

Herbal Teabags Many herbs come ready for use in teabags. To relieve the itch and reduce swelling of teary, watery eyes, apply cold, damp teabags of elder flower, Chinese, or fennel tea to closed eyes as poultices, and relax for ten to fifteen minutes.

Sandalwood and Pine Steam Treatment* To remove excess mucus from nasal passages and ease breathing problems caused by allergy congestion, you might mix fifteen drops of sandalwood oil with fifteen drops of pine oil, and ten drops of lavender oil. Mix the ingredients together in a dark glass bottle (which protects the contents from sunlight and heat) and shake vigorously. Fill a basin with boiling water. Add a teaspoon of the mixture to the water. Lean over the basin with a large towel draped over your head, and inhale the herbal steam for ten minutes. Stay in a warm room for at least thirty minutes after the treatment. Note: Epileptics or those with nerve disorders should avoid using pine oil.

Sandalwood Oil For the relief of congestion, add five drops of sandalwood oil to a bowl of water and place on your bedside table to inhale while you sleep, but keep it out of the reach of children and pets.

*Essential oils are for external use only. This treatment should not be used by children, asthmatics, or those with high blood pressure.

Bayberry Commercially prepared bayberry is useful for reducing secretions and discharge; it may be used as a gargle. To clear up a congested chest, try applying a compress soaked in bayberry solution to your chest at several intervals during the day.

Fenugreek Fenugreek helps break up respiratory mucus. You can take it as a commercially prepared tea twice daily. Fenugreek should not be used if you are pregnant.

Mullein When taken as a commercially prepared tea twice daily, mullein is useful in the treatment of hay fever.

Diet and Nutritional Supplements

The immune system is often taken for granted, although our health is dependent on its proper functioning. In the case of allergies, our immune system especially needs our help if it is to be fueled with the ingredients necessary for our health. Because allergies press the immune system into overactivity, they increase our susceptibility to other ailments.

We can assist the functioning of our immune system by reducing our body's burden of toxic chemicals acquired from poor food choices. The elimination of heavily processed foods, luncheon meats, chicken and turkey injected with chemicals and hormones, sugary snacks, and refined flour products is a good first step to take. In the case of allergic reactions to mold, diet considerations would include avoiding cheese, mushrooms, dried fruits, and soy sauce. Bioflavonoids (found in the pulp, rind, and juice of oranges, lemons, and grapefruit) have an anti-allergy effect and can easily be consumed by cooking strips of orange and lemon peels in a little honey until soft. Eat daily, especially when allergies are at their worst. In addition, you should be sure to consume adequate zinc, omega-3 and omega-6 fatty acids, magnesium, quercetin, and vitamins A, E, and C.

(Note: Vitamin A is toxic if taken in high doses.) Evening primrose oil has been touted for its anti-inflammatory actions and is helpful for fighting congestion.

A nutritionist can help you design a diet that will give your body the proper balance of vitamins and minerals to keep your immune system strong. Food can be useful in other ways as well. Below are tips for using the food in your pantry to treat your allergies:

Miso Soup   A fermented, aged soybean puree, miso soup is a popular item in Japanese restaurants and is also sold at health food stores. It contains enzymes that aid digestion and helps relieve many of the symptoms of allergy.

Horseradish   Horseradish is a great cleanser and stimulant. Mix horseradish with a small amount of apple cider vinegar. Start by taking a quarter teaspoon—slowly increase the amount to a half teaspoon (or your tolerance level)—four times daily to clear congestion. Keep a bowl of horseradish within whiffing distance of your bed at night. You'll sleep like a baby.

Cider Vinegar   Cider vinegar can combat hay fever symptoms. Drink one glass daily of one tablespoon of vinegar mixed with one tablespoon of honey in a glass of water. This is not only good for hay fever, but it is an excellent health tonic as well.

Meditation

Meditation is useful for relieving stress and calming the body and mind. In this highly technological society, we often forget that "in quietness . . . shall be your strength" (Isaiah 30:15). We are constantly on the go, working long hours, eating unbalanced meals, and pushing our bodies to the maximum.

Somewhere in our lives, we need to maintain an oasis of calm to which we can retreat to replenish our vitality and produce a fresh well of energy. If we don't slow down, we face the risk of burnout, and endanger our health in the process. Meditation helps us to maintain an inner core of tranquillity. In turn, calming the body calms the immune system and eliminates some of the oversensitivity to substances that sometimes results in allergies. Stress has been shown to be a factor in weakening the immune system; consequently, a process such as meditation that provides relief from stress will be beneficial in reducing allergy symptoms.

Select and learn a meditation technique that feels comfortable for you. A wide range of books, tapes, videos, and classes is available for learning the various kinds of meditation techniques. One simple meditation technique is to sit in a darkened room with your feet flat on the floor and your hands folded in your lap. Close your eyes and slowly repeat a mantra (a word or phrase) over and over again, in a continuous, soothing rhythm. When thoughts threaten to enter your head, simply ignore them—imagine them as feathers floating slowly away from you—and continue to repeat the mantra many times, using it to focus your attention. Don't feel that you have to work at repeating the mantra; it should be part of the natural flow of things, and you can repeat it as slowly or quickly as you wish. Many people choose the word "one" because it creates a nice vibration and a humming sound when continuously repeated. After about a half hour, you can stop repeating the mantra. Sit quietly for a few minutes to ease yourself slowly out of your meditative state.

Set a goal of meditating at least once a day, either before meals or at least two hours after eating. If you have a hectic schedule, reduce your session from one half hour to fifteen minutes. It's more important to get into the habit of daily practice than to spend a long time, and a short session is better than no session at all. Don't expect to become an instant expert or to obtain results immediately. However, if you practice daily, you should see some results within a few weeks of beginning.

Homeopathic allergy remedies

Homeopathic remedies for allergies are formulated after the homeopathic health care provider has taken an extensive case history. The homeopath will take into consideration your symptoms, how and when they occur, as well as if, when, and why they subside, your personal and family medical history, immunization history, and other factors such as environment and lifestyle. You will be given tablets or drops of a specific remedy designed specially in response to your particular allergies, along with instructions on when and how to administer the remedy. (See chapter 1 for further instructions on homeopathic remedies.) If you think that your remedy is not working after you have used it for a few days, ask the homeopath for another remedy.

Some common homeopathic allergy remedies are:

- *kali bichromicum*—commonly used for treating head congestion
- *arsenicum album*—used for treating allergic symptoms, for example a runny nose
- *pulsitilla*—useful for treating allergies and ear infections, particularly for reducing symptoms of hay fever during an attack
- *sabadilla*—used to treat allergy symptoms such as runny nose, sneezing, and itchy eyes
- *wyethia*—beneficial for allergy sufferers with runny nose, dry throat, or itching in the palate or behind the nose
- *euphrasia*—useful for treating runny nose, watery eyes, and certain kinds of coughs

- *phosphorus*—often works by transforming internal symptoms into external symptoms—for example, pimples may crop up after a successful treatment. The treatment should not be given during hay fever season because it may exaggerate symptoms

Hay fever remedies are available in health food stores and are prepared as solutions in small glass vials, or in the form of dried granules or pills. The bottles are labeled according to the degree of dilution, with higher potencies having been diluted a greater number of times. For example, a 6c solution is not as potent as a 20c solution, which would have been processed twenty times more vigorously in comparison to the 6c solution, which is diluted in a proportion of 1:100 and shaken a mere six times. These formulas are considered safe and nontoxic, but you may prefer to consult a homeopath for a more individualized remedy.

Acupressure

Practitioners of the form of massage called acupressure recognize the connection between physical and mental symptoms. Like acupuncture, acupressure aims to restore and balance body energies and release stress and tension. Some acupressure practitioners integrate breathing meditations into their routines, while others offer herbal remedies. All will work with massage to restore a feeling of relaxation in the body. Specific symptoms (sneezing, nasal congestion, headache, swollen eyes, and head congestion) related to particular allergies can be relieved by applying pressure to points around the skull, nose, and neck area. For more information about specific styles of acupressure, refer to the discussion of acupressure in chapter 3.

Reflexology

Another holistic technique, reflexology applies massage and pressure to points on the feet and hands in order to stimulate different organs in the body. This approach is based on the assumption of correspondences between parts of the feet and the body's various organs. If you were to glance at a reflexology chart, you would notice, for instance, that reflex areas in the feet corresponding to the sinus, head, and brain are located in the region of the toe. The top joints and knuckles of the hands also correspond to the sinus area. A reflexologist will apply direct pressure to these specific points in order to break up deposits of waste material and unblock nerve impulses. Reflexology is as relaxing as a whole body massage; and, an added advantage is that you don't have to fully disrobe in order to reap the benefits.

TREATMENTS FOR HAY FEVER
AND ALLERGIC RHINITIS

Conventional	Alternative
Medications	*Nutrition*
Antihistamines, decongestants, nasal sprays	Zinc, quercetin, omega-3 and omega-6 fatty acids, evening primrose oil, magnesium, vitamins A, E, C
Environmental Changes	*Homeopathy*
Avoidance of allergens	Custom remedies
Immunotherapy (Allergy Shots)	*Acupressure/Reflexology*
Injection of allergen to reduce sensitivity	Pressure applied to specific points
	Herbal Treatments
	Individual remedies

Combination Treatments

So far, no perfect formula for treating allergies has been discovered. Both allopathic and natural medicine stress the avoidance of the allergen whenever possible; however, in the case of some allergens, such as pollen and dust, avoidance can be very difficult to accomplish. Allopathic medicine offers medications to relieve symptoms, while natural medicine offers a wide range of solutions ranging from acupuncture to electromagnetic therapy. Not all of these therapies will work for all people. To provide relief and restore health, most allergy programs require a menu of therapies that fit together like a puzzle. Many individuals will not find a solution until an initial period of trial and error has elapsed. The main thing to remember is that there is no perfect solution, only what is comfortable and right for you. If you feel better and your symptoms have been relieved, then the treatment is working for you.

You have a great number of choices; and although choices can sometimes lead to confusion, integrating allopathic and alternative methods is generally worth the effort. By making the proper environmental change—such as dusting daily with a damp cloth, controlling the humidity in your home and keeping windows closed to keep out pollen—you can limit exposure to your allergen. Once you have made those basic changes, you can use allopathic medications to control symptoms, and you can adjust your diet to support your immune system. Bodywork techniques such as acupressure and reflexology will relax your body, release energy and ease organ blockages, all of which may help to reduce stress during peak allergy seasons. Here are some other tips for your integrated treatment plan:

- Take stinging nettle capsules as part of a preventive care program for hay fever.

- Use essential oils in steam treatments.
- Bathe each night to avoid bringing allergens into bed with you.
- Consider immunotherapy if other techniques don't bring relief.
- Learn about herbs and use them to relieve allergy-related stuffy noses, sore throats, and headaches.
- Eliminate food additives and preservatives from your diet. Eat a balanced diet that avoids allergy-triggering foods, drink lots or water, and keep your weight down. The less baggage you have the better you'll feel.
- Support the body's immune systems with vitamin C and other supplements.
- Use antihistamines or nose sprays to clear congestion, or take appropriate herbal hay-fever products approved by your doctor.

CHAPTER 5

Skin Allergies and Eczema

The skin is our largest organ of elimination. It is like our third lung—it breathes and removes toxic wastes through the tiniest of pores. These toxins are often the cause of skin allergies, rashes, and hives. What exactly is a skin allergy? The term covers a broad spectrum of conditions, symptoms, and triggers, although the three most common conditions are contact dermatitis, hives, and eczema.

Hives usually appear in the form of itchy red patches called wheals. They are unattractive, annoying, and usually harmless; they can be brought about by a number of factors, ranging from cold weather to medications such as penicillin. If you can discover the cause of your hives, then you can take precautions to prevent further outbreaks. Some people, however, try to treat themselves and end up smothering their hives with heavy creams or lotions that can harm their skin and cause further irritation. Hives can also develop from hidden food allergies, which is one reason why it is best to get at the root of the problem; what shows up on your skin is a good indication of what is going on inside your body.

Another common skin allergy, called eczema, or atopic dermatitis, is a chronic skin disease that tends to be most common in people who suffer from other allergies, such as hay fever or food allergies. As in the case of hives, it is best to get to the root of the problem, for the sake not only of your skin but of your general health. Supplements such as evening primrose oil, which will be discussed later in the chapter, often work wonders in clearing up eczema when taken daily, demonstrating that it is what you put in your body rather than on your skin that affects it most.

Contact dermatitis is perhaps the easiest to resolve since it is purely an external condition. The only way to cure a case of contact dermatitis is to eliminate prolonged contact with the allergen that you are treating. The major challenge is to pinpoint the substance causing the allergic reaction, and a good health care provider can do the proper detective work to do this.

Everyone wants healthy, soft, clear skin: we are not at our best with itchy, red, raw skin. If you are suffering from hives, eczema, or contact dermatitis, your skin is probably affecting your confidence and self-esteem. So it is important to get to the root of the problem and treat it as soon as possible.

GETTING TO THE ROOT OF HIVES

Hives are round, red, extremely itchy, swollen areas of skin. They seem to come from nowhere, popping up suddenly and then disappearing within hours or days. They tend to appear on arms, legs, or any exposed area, often in clusters. Hives spring from a wide variety of sources. They can be caused by an adverse reaction to a food or drug, or even an insect sting. Swallowing ice cubes or cold drinks can provoke a hive on the lips or mouth. Foods such as peanuts, milk, fish, eggs, tomatoes, and berries are also common causes of hives. Medications such as penicillin, sulfa, and anticonvulsant drugs, as well as aspirin, can provoke hives. Hives resulting either from heat from a fever, a hot tub, or shower, or from strong emotions and stress are referred to as *cholinergic urticaria*. Such factors as cold wind and water can account for *cold-induced urticaria*, while strong sunlight can often result in an outbreak of hives known as *solar urticaria*. Hives can also result from chronic candidiasis, an infection caused by an overgrowth of *Candida albicans*—a yeast normally found in the vagina, on skin, and in the intestinal tract that poses little threat to our health if maintained at normal levels. But such factors as an impaired immune system, overuse of antibiotics, anti-inflammatory drugs, and immunosuppressive drugs can make it possible for the yeast to accumulate and create trouble. If there is an overgrowth of candida in the system, hives can appear on the skin.

In the treatment of hives, avoidance of the food, drugs, or other allergens to which an individual is oversensitive is highly recommended. Never underestimate the power of hives. Hives on the mouth and throat can be life-threatening by blocking breathing passages. Severe, acute hives should always receive the attention of a physician.

ALLERGIC ECZEMA

Allergic eczema, often referred to as dermatitis, is an inflammation of the skin, with symptoms such as blistering, red bumps, swelling, crusting, and unsightly scaling. The causes are wide-ranging, but some of the most common factors are food and other allergies, nutritional deficiencies in vitamin B, and stress. Eczema can be controlled; contrary to public misunderstanding, it is not contagious.

Here are the various types of eczema:

- *Contact eczema* results from irritants, allergic substances, light, chemicals, or perfume.

- *Atopic eczema* occurs in people with asthma and allergy problems or with B12 deficiency. Infants two to eighteen months old usually develop a rash, red spots on the face, scalp, or extremities. Breast-fed children are less likely to have eczema, so if you want to prevent eczema in your children, breast-feed!
- *Seborrheic dermatitis,* or eczema, often appears on the scalp, face, and chest areas.
- *Nummular dermatitis,* or eczema, is characterized by coin-shaped red spots that crust and scale. It is usually chronic and occurs after thirty-five years of age. It is associated with stress and dry skin.
- *Chronic eczema* is found on hands and feet and can become very severe. Latex allergy may also cause eczema; it is named for the milky sap collected from the rubber tree, which is used in such products as household gloves, condoms, bandages, and baby-bottle nipples.
- *Generalized eczema* is spread over much of the body's skin surface.
- *Statis eczema* is found in the lower leg area and is associated with poor circulation.
- *Localized scratch eczema* occurs in specific patches. It is often marked by whitish areas and is aggravated by stress and scratching.

Certain allergens or irritants, such as the following, that should be suspected in eczema:

- Common irritants include soap, shampoo, wool, household chemicals, solvents, heat, and excessive scratching.
- Common food suspects in cases of eczema are milk, eggs, and citrus fruits. Chicken, nuts, wheat, fish, toma-

toes and soya, food additives, and preservatives are also commonly related to eczema. To learn more about how food allergies affect the body, refer to chapter 6 on food allergies.

- Metals found in jewelry and other products are common offenders and the most frequently cited ones are nickel, chromium, and cobalt.

CONTACT DERMATITIS

It begins shortly after you buy a new bar of that fancy soap you'd been wanting to try—the soap that costs a small fortune and promises clear, smooth skin that feels like velvet. But instead of the clear, smooth skin promised by the advertisement, you break out in clusters of ugly red bumps that appear to be hives. Most likely, you've developed an allergic reaction known as contact dermatitis, resulting from prolonged contact with an allergen. It is a localized reaction, confined to the area that is directly exposed to the allergen. This means that if you are allergic to dishwashing liquid—a common cause of contact dermatitis—the rash would be confined to your hands. Any number of substances can be involved, but the most common offenders are hair dyes and cosmetics, earrings and bracelets, glasses, clothing, chemicals, rubber, detergents, plants, aftershave, and shaving cream. The only solution is the removal of the allergen. Once the allergen is removed, the rash will disappear.

Traditional Treatments

Because allergies are so complex and each case has its own triggers and symptoms, it is difficult to predict what results you will get from testing and treatment.

Hives and eczema can come and go so quickly that many people never get tested at all. That's a shame, because they might discover that the roots of the condition often lie in far more complex health problems, such as food allergies. Most cases of skin allergy are usually not life-threatening; however, special precautions must be taken with hives located around the mouth area, since acute cases can interfere with breathing and swallowing, and can even be fatal.

If you have a skin rash or a case of hives that is persistent or particularly troubling, you should see a doctor who specializes in skin conditions immediately. During your office visit, the doctor will closely examine your skin to determine what kind of rash it is and then ask you questions for clues about what caused it. Once the source of the rash has been discovered, the health care provider can prescribe a course of treatment.

In the case of contact dermatitis a patch test will be used to determine the source of the allergy. A small pad containing a possible allergen will be taped onto your back and the result should be apparent in two days. While you are wearing the pad, you will be asked to avoid wetting that area and told not to engage in vigorous activities such as sports or exercise. If you experience any pain or unusually severe itching during this period, call your health care provider. Once the patch is removed and the area has been evaluated, a diagnosis is made, and treatment of the allergy can begin.

Avoidance

Eliminating or avoiding the allergen is the primary method of dealing with most skin allergies. You will be instructed to avoid extremes of temperature, chemicals, dust, and solvents, and to avoid scratching your skin once it has become inflamed. Those with contact dermatitis should take precautions such as wearing rubber gloves with cotton liners while performing household chores. People with eczema, who are very prone to the temptation to scratch their inflamed skin, should trim their fingernails closely in case they can't resist. They must avoid substances including harsh detergents, soap, wool, any prickly fabrics, and tight clothing, that irritate and scratch the skin. If you have eczema, you should cleanse your fragile skin with gentle cleansers such as glycerin and rosewater and apply lanolin-free skin moisturizers frequently. Other measures include avoiding extreme temperatures as well as activities that cause excessive sweating or stress. Your health care provider may recommend taking baths with special nonprescription skin treatments—ask for recommendations—to ease itching.

Epinephrine and Emergency Room Treatment

As discussed earlier in this chapter, skin allergies are not merely unattractive: They can under certain circumstances require emergency room visits and even be fatal as well. Hives located in the mouth or throat area can block breathing passages and cause death. If you have difficulty breathing, go to an emergency room *immediately*. If you have chronic hives or if they are severe, speak to your doctor about prescribing epinephrine for emergency use. Epinephrine is a synthetic version of adrenaline that saves lives by reversing throat swelling, relaxing lung muscles, and stimulating heartbeat. To learn more about epinephrine, refer to chapter 2 on adult asthma.

Medications

There is a wide array of medication available for skin allergies and symptoms. External remedies for skin allergies include over-the-counter astringents, hydrocortisone, calamine lotion, and zinc oxide to relieve itching. Consult your doctor for the medication best suited to your particular condition.

Alternative Treatments
The alternative practitioner will view factors such as heredity, diet, environment, lifestyle, and emotions as clues for understanding the development of skin allergies. Different explanations lead to different treatments, and while some will work for you, others won't. Experimenting is the only way to find out, and in the process you may come closer to discovering what does trigger your allergies.

We all know how stress can affect the body. Anyone who has made it through the teen years can attest to the fact that a pimple is a thousand times likelier to appear on your face the day before the senior prom or a major test than on just an ordinary day. There is no question that stress can affect the skin and aggravate eczema and hives. Alternative therapies have much to offer in the way of mind-body approaches, which more and more allopathic health care providers are finally beginning to accept. The use of hydrotherapy, for instance, to relax the body and mind and the use of essential oils and mixtures to soothe the skin are based on a holistic approach to resolving skin allergies.

Other alternative approaches, such as using herbs to cleanse and detoxify the body, incorporate natural elements into our chemical-laden lives. Herbal formulas are comfortable and easy to use, and you'll enjoy mixing a recipe for soothing, natural relief, as you'll discover in this chapter.

Hydrotherapy

Hydrotherapy relieves stress, improves circulation, and rids the body of toxins; and it is often recommended by an alternative health care practitioner or osteopathic health care provider as part of a broader treatment plan. Although there are many elaborate methods of adding hydrotherapy to your life, taking a healing bath in your home is one simple yet excellent way to treat skin allergies and release tension in a familiar and comfortable environment. You may add essential oils, but use the lowest recommended dosage or reduce by half if you have sensitive skin, and don't use at all if you are pregnant; you may also add herbs to soothe irritated skin, relieve itching, and remove toxins from the body.

There are some precautions you should take, however, when using essential oils or herbs in your bath. A primary health care provider should always be consulted before any herb is used, particularly in the case of pregnant women, children, or people who have certain medical conditions or are using medications. In any case, do not use any herb or essential oil for a prolonged period of time, combine them on your own, or use them in large doses. Some herbs can be toxic even in small doses, so never use a herb you are unfamiliar with or know little about. Be alert for any adverse reactions or side effects, which you should immediately discuss with your primary health care provider. Note: Asthmatics should check with their health care provider before using essential oils.

Below are some recommended baths:

- *Apple cider vinegar* removes toxins, relieves poison ivy, and restores the natural covering essential for maintaining healthy skin. Add one cup to a lukewarm tub of water.
- *Cornstarch* helps to reduce itchiness caused by eczema. One pound can be mixed with one or two cups of col-

loidal oatmeal (available in drugstores) for additional soothing and restoration of the skin.

- *Baking soda* relieves skin irritation and itching. Add one pound to your bath.
- *Chamomile* is an herb that may soothe eczema and hives. Add a few drops to bath water.
- *Jasmine oil* is a beneficial remedy for treating eczema and other skin allergies. Add five drops to your bath water.
- *Lemon oil* is very effective in relieving the itchiness of many skin allergies. Add five drops to your bath, while symptoms persist, after checking with your health care provider. Do not use for a prolonged period of time.
- *Salt* removes toxins from the body. Add one pound to a warm tub of water.
- *Honey* has been used to soothe wounds since biblical times. A few drops of honey added to the bath will soothe and nourish tender skin.
- *Pine oil* softens the skin and relieves rashes. Add five drops to your bath. Do not use if you have high blood pressure, and always consult a health care provider before using essential oils as part of a personal treatment program. Note: Epileptics or those with nerve disorders should avoid using pine oil.

Herbal Treatments

Herbal treatments release toxins, reduce symptoms, and soothe irritated and inflamed skin. Although it may take some experimenting before you hit on the appropriate solution, it can be worth the effort. However, always consult your primary health care provider before using herbal remedies. You might also consult a botanical practitioner who will meet with you several times to discuss your symptoms and create a specialized treatment program. Depending on such a specialist's findings, herbs will be prescribed to detoxify, nourish, cleanse, calm, warm, or cool your system.

As indicated above, you should not prepare your own remedies, and you should keep in mind that in the case of children, pregnant women, or people with a medical condition such as high blood pressure, special precautions must be taken. Remember: no herb should be used for a prolonged period of time, and you should not combine herbs on your own or use any herb in large doses. Always be alert for any adverse reactions or side effects, which you should immediately discuss with your primary health care provider.

The following herbs have been helpful in treating skin allergies:

Burdock Commercially prepared burdock is often used to treat such skin conditions as eczema, rashes, and hives; it can be applied externally to heal skin eruptions. But be warned: the growing plant may actually cause contact dermatitis.

Black Currant Oil The oil from black currants is an excellent anti-inflammatory agent. Apply externally to treat skin allergies.

Black Walnut Black walnut is especially good for treating eczema. The commercially prepared herb can be used internally and externally.

Evening Primrose Oil The external seed oil of the evening primrose can be applied externally to soften dry, scaly, itchy skin.

Calendula (Pot Marigold) The herbal cream derived from the Calendula, or pot marigold, can be applied externally to soothe cracked, dry, and painful skin. Calendula creams and lotions can be purchased in many health-food stores.

Chickweed   You can mix one to two cups of chickweed tea in your bath to relieve itching.

Golden Seal   Golden seal belongs to the buttercup family; it grows in warm climates. The commercially prepared herb can be applied externally to assist in treating eczema. It should not be used if you suffer from high blood pressure or are pregnant.

Oregon Grape   The Oregon grape is especially helpful as a remedy for chronic eczema. It can be taken as a commercially prepared tea or used externally by placing its liquid or oil on a wet, hot compress and applying it to the affected area.

Yellow Dock   Yellow dock is a cleansing herb and a tonic for the treatment of eczema and other skin allergies. Do not use it to excess, as large amounts can cause diarrhea.

Red Clover   Taken internally, commercially prepared red clover soothes the frazzled nerves that can contribute to skin allergies. It is excellent for treating eczema because it purifies the blood. Do not give this herb to children, the elderly, or pregnant women.

Homeopathy

Homeopathy frowns on the use of products such as calamine lotion and hydrocortisone, which are viewed, at best, as ways of masking symptoms and, at worst, of causing significant imbalances in the body. Although a homeopathic practitioner will initially advise avoidance of the allergen as the best form of treatment, he or she also can administer natural, nontoxic remedies to help the body recover from allergies and to ease symptoms until recovery is complete. Be sure to store your homeopathic remedies in the original container and keep them away from strong light, temperatures, and scents. Don't keep the container open for long, and try not to touch the rim of the bottle. For more guidelines on the proper way to administer your homeopathic remedy, refer to the discussion of homeopathy in chapter 2 on adult asthma.

Following are a couple of common homeopathic remedies for treating skin allergies:

- *rhus tox icodendron* is used for treating contact dermatitis and other allergy symptoms, including burning, itching, and oozing blisters.
- *apis* is useful for treating itchy hives.

Diet and Nutrition

An alternative health care practitioner will usually treat skin problems such as eczema and hives by addressing your diet. Of course, in the case of contact dermatitis, common sense dictates that external allergens such as jewelry, clothing, bedding, or other sources of skin irritation be removed and avoided.

Eczema and hives are often caused by food allergies and poor diet habits. The alternative health care practitioner might initially prescribe an elimination diet (see chapter 6) to determine if food allergies are at the root of the problem. You will start off on a diet of foods that are unlikely to provoke an allergic response and then slowly add additional foods. Meanwhile, your body has had time to eliminate toxins and begin to heal. If any foods gradually being reintroduced into your diet cause an allergic reaction, those substances will have to be removed. Further dietary changes might include the addition of omega-3 fatty oils—good sources are sardines, salmon, herring, mackerel, tuna, and the fish oil supplement Max EPA found in health food stores—as well as vitamins A, C, E, B complex, magnesium, and zinc. Evening primrose oil is another important supplement to help normalize the digestion of fatty acids, which may be a problem for people suffering from eczema.

Eggs, milk, and citrus fruits are common dietary offenders (especially in the case of eczema) and are tested as possible allergens. If they test positive, they will be removed from the diet. The addition of friendly bacteria in the form of lactobacillus may also be necessary, particularly in the case of individuals who also have yeast infections. The best method of adding this friendly bacteria is in the form of daily servings of cultured dairy products such as yogurt; or if you are sensitive to milk, you can purchase concentrated capsules with guaranteed potency at your health-food or drugstore. Before purchasing anything, be sure to check for a bacteriological analysis showing the number of live bacteria per gram. Look for capsules containing several million bacteria per gram.

The case of Marsha provides an excellent example of the importance of diet in treating allergies. Marsha had gone to a medical health care provider who had told her that she had urticaria (hives) and that she was allergic to strawberries, nuts, wheat, soybeans, and pork. He put her on an allergy diet and eliminated all of the foods to which she was allergic. Her symptoms improved slightly—about 10 percent—leaving Marsha and her health care provider a bit perplexed. They couldn't understand why her improvement was so slight. Unhappy with her condition, Marsha sought out an alternative health care provider whose physical examination revealed hives on her chest, back, arms, and buttocks, especially under the elastic borders of her underclothes. Her routine blood studies were normal, as were her permeability and liver tests. A vital clue was finally uncovered when her comprehensive digestive stool analysis (CDSA) revealed a massive candida invasion. She had a yeast infection without knowing it. Allergies to certain foods can be worse if you are infected with yeast. Eliminating the allergic foods is not enough, as you can see in Marsha's case. Her yeast infection was cleared up with supplements such as Nutri Stattin 144, Aller Clear, and Hepatox (all by BioMetrics). She was also given vitamin C supplements and Cal-Mag Citrate, which can be found in health food stores or at Hickey Chemist Ltd., at 888 Second Avenue, New York City (telephone: (800) 724-5566). Marsha was put on a yeast-free diet, which meant eliminating the following:

- most B-vitamin preparations (except B complex)
- vinegars and products containing vinegar
- fermented beverages such as alcohol and ginger ale
- baked goods raised with baker's yeast
- foods high in mold content such as aged cheeses, buttermilk, and sour cream or yogurt
- citrus juices, unless home squeezed
- monosodium glutamate (MSG) and citric acid, which are yeast derivatives
- dried fruits
- grapes and grape juices
- refined carbohydrates, which means refined flour and white sugar
- mushrooms

Clearing up candida is one thing. Keeping it from coming back is another, especially if you revert to your old eating habits. Try to eat as little sugar and refined carbohydrates as you possibly can. If your symptoms return, have your health care provider test you again: You may have to go back on a restricted, yeast-free diet for a while.

Reflexology

You walk into a darkened room, slip your shoes off, and relax while the reflexologist skillfully works on your tender feet. Stress slips away as the practitioner works to correct the buildup of toxins in the body that reflexologists believe to be the cause of skin allergies. Your reflexology session for the treatment of skin allergies will include work on the reflex points that correspond to the kidneys, liver, adrenal glands, thyroid, and lymphatic systems. Although your skin problems will not be immediately resolved, you will leave each session feeling more relaxed, which will help to reduce any symptoms that you are experiencing as the result of stress.

Keep in mind that reflexology is not a cure-all and that you will have to do some work in other areas as well. However, combined with changes in your diet and homeopathic or herbal treatment, a reflexology program that is approved by your primary health care practitioner may be useful in reducing the severity and frequency of skin allergies.

Acupressure

Acupressure treatments are another way to attack the stress that lies at the root of many skin allergies. During an acupressure session for the treatment of skin allergies, the practitioner will use the body's pressure points to relieve stress and increase circulation. In addition, the practitioner will concentrate on specific points to stimulate the corresponding organs and glands that are essential to maintaining healthy skin. Tonic points located in the lower back will be massaged in order to stimulate the immune system. Some practitioners may want you to concentrate on your breathing, and will teach you how to use your full lung capacity. You may also need to conjure up your full powers of concentration to focus on the life force flowing in and out of the affected areas of your skin as the practitioner works on your body. Feel the release of tension and visualize it flowing away and out of your system. Visualize your skin getting stronger as the practitioner places direct pressure on the toxins in your system.

You may want to book weekly or biweekly sessions for a few months, even attending these sessions after all symptoms are gone as part of a holistic treatment plan for your allergies. However, although acupressure is effective in relieving stress and improving circulation, it is not meant to replace treatment by a health care provider and it should be used only as part of a total treatment program.

Meditation

Stress is recognized as a factor in skin allergies such as hives and eczema. It can hinder the function of the immune system, a condition known as immunosuppression, making the body more vulnerable to illness. As an adjunct to more traditional forms of medicine, meditation offers a chemical-free immune system booster that may aid in the management of allergies. It is beneficial in reducing stress levels and thus creating the proper environment for other therapies to perform effectively and help you heal.

There are many types of meditation, ranging from Transcendental Meditation to walking meditation. You can pay as little as $10 for a meditation tape or as much as $500 for a meditation course. Finding out which method works best for you may involve some experimentation. However, all types of meditation have basic premises that anyone can grasp. Try to sit quietly in a chair or cross-legged on the floor of a dimly lit room, with your back straight and your hands resting on your knees. Learning to breathe for relaxation is essential. Your breathing must be steady, deep, and rhythmic. Your abdomen should expand and deflate as you inhale and exhale. A word or phrase (such as the word *one*) that is continuously repeated while you meditate is known as a *mantra*. A mantra provides a focus during meditation and may have a somewhat hypnotic effect, allowing your mind to clear and relaxation to set in.

Whatever type of meditation you choose to do, remember that it takes a while to develop the skill to focus fully, let your cares float away, and "let it go." When you do reach that state, your tension and stress will be much reduced.

TREATMENTS FOR SKIN ALLERGIES AND ECZEMA

Conventional	Alternative
Medications Antihistamines, calamine lotion, zinc oxide, hydrocortisone cream	**Homeopathy** Customized remedies
	Hydrotherapy Essential oils, herbs, salts
Environmental Changes Avoidance and removal of allergens	**Herbal Treatments** Commercially prepared teas, external creams, compresses
	Diet and Nutritional Supplements Omega-3 fatty oils, vitamin A, E, B-complex, vitamin C, zinc, magnesium, evening primrose oil, Nutri Stattin 144, Aller Clear, Hepatox

Combined Treatments

Because treating allergies is not an exact science, trial and error is required in any course of treatment. Not every therapy will work for each person, but there is enough of a range of options to offer relief and attack the roots of the problem. If skin allergies are acute and life-threatening, allopathic medications and technology can bring significant relief. In more moderate to mild allergic conditions, alternative therapies can be a useful adjunct in treatment, combined with allopathic medicine for optimum benefit. Among the possible combinations are the integration of herbal remedies—with your primary health care practitioner—into your total treatment program to relieve symptoms and cleanse toxins, and the use of bodywork treatments, such as acupressure and reflexology to support the body's healing process, during allopathic medical treatment. Other alternative therapies that can complement an allopathic treatment plan for the sake of your skin are:

- nutritional supplements such as evening primrose oil, omega-3 fatty acids, zinc, magnesium, and vitamin C to build skin health from the inside out
- meditation to relieve the stress that can cause skin conditions to worsen or develop in the first place
- hydrotherapy treatments consisting of essential oils and other products

CHAPTER 6

Food Allergies

Food nourishes our bodies and our souls. When we sit down at a pleasantly decorated table and we are stimulated by the fragrant aromas and the vibrant colors and shapes, we relax and enjoy our meal, knowing that the food will satisfy our hunger, replenish our energy, and maintain our health. *Unless something goes wrong.* Seemingly out of the blue, your eyes may begin to tear. Your stomach may turn gassy and bloated. Could it be food poisoning—or flu? You're not sure, but you do know that lately after you eat certain foods that have been your favorites for a long time, you don't come away with a pleasurable sensation. Instead, you experience heartburn, gas, nausea, and pain. What's even more confusing is that you're constantly craving the food that your body seems to reject. What on earth is going on? You've been breaking out in rashes. You feel dizzy and tired and even a bit sad at times, and you can't understand why. And you still have those food cravings—for cheesecake, bread, and anything made with flour or wheat. If you suffer from these perplexing and complex symptoms, there's a good possibility that you have a food allergy.

Although many people think that they suffer from food allergies, experts estimate that only 2 percent of adults and 2 to 8 percent of children are truly allergic to foods. Food intolerance—see chapter 7 for further details—can produce similar symptoms and is much more common. So how do you determine if you suffer from food allergies or food sensitivity? Although these symptoms are not exclusive to food allergy, you may want to see a doctor if you have one or more of the following symptoms:

- dark circles under the eyes
- feeling of fullness in the head; headaches
- runny or stuffy nose, excess mucus, postnasal drip, watery eyes
- sore throat, hoarseness, gagging, recurrent sinusitis
- mucus in stools, nausea, vomiting, diarrhea, constipation, belching
- extreme thirst, irritable bowel syndrome, cramps
- weakness, muscle aches, swellings of the hands, feet, and ankles
- cravings, binge eating, rapid weight gain

Many factors, including heredity and intestinal permeability, contribute to the development of food allergies. In general, the intestinal tract works as a barrier against the excessive absorption of bacteria and food antigens, any substances that under unfavorable conditions stimulate the production of antibodies. When this digestive mechanism is altered by factors such as aging, infection, or trauma, antigens are allowed to enter the system in excessive amounts, leading to increased sensitivity and a potential immune response to food. Although it may seem as if food allergy is restricted to the digestive tract, air passages, and skin, food allergens that enter the bloodstream can produce a wide range of physical and mental symptoms. That is why it is so important to get a proper diagnosis.

Another reason why we must take food allergies very seriously is the possibility of developing the severe allergic reaction known as anaphylaxis. This potentially deadly allergic reaction was first described in 2641 B.C., on a tablet detailing the death of the Egyptian ruler Menes after he was stung by an insect. Today, hundreds of lives continue to be taken every year by violent reactions to allergens. On exposure to an allergen, symptoms of anaphylaxis can begin in as little as five minutes, and they include swelling of the mouth, throat, and vocal cords, a drop in blood pressure, and loss of consciousness. Breathing and swallowing are severely impaired. The allergic person must be rushed to the emergency room as quickly as possible. Every second counts. Later in this chapter we will describe the use of epinephrine, a form of adrenaline that can and does save lives. Epinephrine works directly on the cardiovascular and respiratory systems, reversing swelling, relaxing lung muscles, and stimulating the heartbeat.

FOOD ADDITIVE ALLERGIES

Many people suffer from allergies to food additives and preservatives that are quite common in many of the foods we consume every day. The following is a list of common food additives that have been known to cause allergic reactions ranging from mild to life-threatening.

Aspartame   Aspartame (brand name NutraSweet) is not an allergen, yet many people suffer adverse reactions to it. It is used as a low-calorie sweetener in desserts, sodas, gum and other foods. People who are particularly sensitive to aspartame are individuals with the genetic disease phenylketonuria (PKU) (inability to absorb the amino acid phenylalanine), individuals with advanced liver disease, and pregnant women with high levels of phenylalanine in the blood.

BHT/BHA   BHT/BHA, an additive that slows the development of food odors, color changes, and off-flavors by preserving oxygen absorption, may occasionally cause hives. It is usually found in high-fat foods and oils, as a preservative in bread, milk, mayonnaise, soft drinks, and instant drinks, and is also used to preserve grain.

Monosodium Glutamate (MSG)   Best known as "Chinese restaurant syndrome" because it is a common ingredient in many Chinese and other Asian dishes, MSG is also used in a variety of processed foods—pickles, soups, candy—including many restaurant foods. It has been known to trigger asthma symptoms, produce hives in some people, and cause headaches.

Nitrate/Nitrites   Used to enhance flavor, color, and preserve foods, nitrate/nitrites are most commonly found in hot dogs, delicatessen meats, and ham. Symptoms range from headaches and vomiting to hives and blood disorders.

Parabens   One of the most frequently used preservatives in the United States, the main function of parabens is to control the growth of molds and yeast in foods. They are generally considered safe; however, some people experience allergic reactions affecting the skin, such as redness, swelling, burning, and itching. Parabens are used in baked goods, sugar substitutes, soft drinks, meat, poultry, fats, oils, among other foods.

Sulfites   Although most people have no problem with sulfites, they are perhaps one of the most potent offenders of all the food additives. Sulfites can cause mild to severe problems for certain people, particularly asthmatics. The FDA categorizes an adverse reaction to sulfites as an "allergic-type response," which can range from mild to life-threatening. The FDA also describes a range of symptoms, such as diarrhea and rashes, suffered by certain individuals after eating sulfite-treated foods.

Sulfites are used primarily as antioxidants, to prevent or reduce discoloration in fruits and vegetables, but they can also be found in such products as wine or beer. You might be surprised to learn that sulfites are also used in the production of cellophane, which is used in food packaging. Sulfites are listed in different ways on food labels: sulfur dioxide, sodium sulfite, sodium and potassium bisulfite, and sodium and potassium metabisulfite. Read your food labels carefully. If you are dining out, ask your server to check if sulfites are used in the meal that you plan to order.

FD & C Yellow No. 5   Listed as tartrazine on medicine labels, FD&C Yellow No. 5 may cause itching or hives in a small number of people. It is also known to provoke migraines and asthmatic attacks. The FDA requires all products containing FD&C Yellow No. 5 to indicate this additive on labels, and you will usually find it in candies, dry cereals, some medicines, and many, but not all, products that are colored yellow or green.

ORAL ALLERGY SYNDROME

Oral allergy syndrome (OAS) is an allergic condition caused by cross-reacting or identical allergens that are present in both a fresh food and a pollen. Common offenders are raw vegetables (carrots, celery, parsley, potatoes, tomatoes), nuts (hazelnuts), seeds (sunflower seeds), or fresh fruits such as apples, apricots, bananas, cantaloupes, cherries, honeydew, oranges, peaches, pears, and watermelon. An oral-allergy syndrome cross-reaction can occur when, for example, you eat an orange on a lawn laden with pollen. The combination of the orange and the pollen create a cross-reaction, such as swelling of the lips, tongue, mouth, or throat, which will usually go away without being treated.

Oral allergy syndrome is always concentrated in the area of the lips, mouth, and throat. It is generally not life-threatening, but, if there is ever any doubt about whether a person's symptoms are due to OAS or anaphylaxis, it is better to err on the safe side and get immediate medical treatment.

LEAKY GUT SYNDROME

Leaky gut syndrome has been linked to the formation of food allergies in certain people. A chronic irritation of the intestinal lining, this syndrome leads to the malabsorption of crucial nutrients. The increased passage of undigested food particles due to a leaky gut creates toxicity and weakens the immune response, leading to increased vulnerability to further allergies. In other words, when your body is absorbing substances that should have been eliminated in the feces and urine, the body becomes bogged down in toxic waste and begins to have trouble digesting food; this can lead to an immune allergic response. In a sense it is a vicious cycle:

- Irritations such as food allergies lead to leaky gut
- Leaky gut leads to the development of more allergies

In an article in *The Lancet* titled "Food Allergy—or Enterometabolic Disorder?" Dr. J. O. Hunter makes the point that although food allergy is thought of as an immune disease, it may actually be more of an "enterometabolic disorder," and he suggests that treatment concentrating on bacterial manipulation to correct food intolerance might be the wave of the future. Extensive work still needs to be done, particularly in understanding gastrointestinal enzyme concentrations, in order to substantiate this hypothesis. However, Hunter feels that factors such as a genetic predisposition toward food allergies, which often runs in families, might actually indicate a predisposition toward a disorder of bacterial fermentation in the colon that itself can lead to food allergies.

The case of a thirty-five-year-old female named Gloria provides a good example of the colon playing a major role in food allergies. Gloria had a fifteen-year history of low energy, weakness, and poor stamina, and all of her symptoms were exacerbated by eating. It didn't seem to matter what she ate, or didn't eat; food of any sort made her condition worse. One doctor told her that she had "global food allergies" which meant that she was allergic to a variety of foods. It was true that as a child she'd had many food allergies, especially to wheat, chocolate, milk, eggs, and dairy. As she got older, her situation worsened, and by the time she was in college her symptoms were so severe that she had to drop out of school. Traditional medical cures had not helped her, nor had the alternative treatments she tried.

After what seemed to be endless testing, a functional liver detoxification profile and an intestinal permeability test finally provided some valuable clues. The functional liver detoxification profile revealed that Gloria was a "pathological detoxifier," which means that the stages involved in her liver detoxification were not following normal patterns. That fact alone could account for her chronic fatigue, since her body was not being properly cleared of toxins. The results of her intestinal permeability tests were just as impressive. She was suffering from leaky gut syndrome. Both of these factors— "pathological detoxification" and "leaky gut syndrome"—were responsible for her long history of allergies and fatigue. She was put on a program of the following nutrients:

- Prodophilus Complex Powder I, II, and III, consisting of super acidophilus culture, L bulgaricus, and bifi-dobacteria-bifidum. One-quarter teaspoon of each was taken daily in three ounces of water, ten minutes before breakfast for three to six months; L-Glutamine Intestinal Permeability Powder: three teaspoons daily (5,000 mgs) were given to normalize intestinal absorption. Both are available from Primary Neutraceuticals by calling 1(800) 839-6554.

- Bio Detox Powder, made by the Institute of Rehabilitative Nutrition (IRN): Two teaspoons daily were taken in water or juice to help increase the ability of the liver to detoxify. You can purchase this product by writing to Institute of Rehabilitative Nutrition, P.O. Box 20199, Columbus Circle Station, New York, NY 10023.

- GHS 250 Master Glutathione Formula, made by Douglas Laboratories, available at health-food stores.

- A multiple antioxidant by Solgar, available at health-food and drug stores.

LIVER DETOXIFICATION AND FOOD ALLERGY

You can't live without your liver. The liver does all of the body's essential dirty work, neutralizing and converting toxins into by-products that are then eliminated. Sometimes we throw a monkey wrench into the system by overchallenging it with chemicals, food allergens, and other toxins. When there is some hitch in the liver detoxification process, we become more vulnerable to illness because the liver ceases to break down toxins effectively or to filter out impurities. A sluggish liver that does not fully detoxify the body is a common problem in cases of food allergy, as was the case with Michael, who appeared in the doctor's office complaining of severe headaches that he had been experiencing for the past fifteen to twenty years. His headaches began everyday at about 4 P.M. and lasted until his head hit the pillow. He'd wake up fatigued, though without any pain. This cycle continued for years, during which time he'd been put through a battery of tests that included head, neck, and sinus X rays, EKG strips, numerous blood and urine tests, and even a spinal tap. None of the tests had succeeded in revealing the source of his head pain. His doctors had prescribed painkillers and told him to exercise more and learn to live with the pain.

The problem was finally solved one day when Michael was given further laboratory tests; all of them tested normal with the exception of the functional liver detoxification profile. It revealed that his liver was sluggish and wasn't fully detoxifying his body, which, as we have seen, is a common cause of food allergies. Michael's diet, unfortunately, consisted of lots of junk foods. In addition, his lunch was usually the same: tuna fish and tomatoes chopped together with hard-boiled eggs. This particular sandwich had been a favorite of his since childhood—it's what his father had eaten for lunch daily. Allergy testing revealed allergies to chocolate, tomatoes, and eggs. Rarely do we see a case that is so clear-cut. Michael was eating his allergenic foods on a daily basis—no wonder he suffered from headaches! The offending foods were removed from his diet and replaced with a variety of other foods. And because his health care provider suspected that he also suffered from hypoglycemia, his meals were spaced at two- to two-and-a-half-hour intervals. Special supplements were added to his diet for liver detoxification and adrenal support. As a result, Michael's headaches were completely gone. All that was left was his craving for sweets. He's still working on that.

Traditional Treatments

If you suspect that you have a food allergy, you should go directly to a doctor who is experienced in this medical specialty. Check to see if the physician has had intensive specialty training in allergy and immunology. Keeping a food diary before your visit is a good first step. For a two-week period before your appointment jot down every single meal, snack, or nibble that you consume and the exact time of day that you eat it. Make a special note of any cravings that you have, because they can provide strong clues and be very helpful in tracking down the cause of food allergies. Do you crave chocolate? Pastries? Wheat products? Peanuts? Peanut butter? What about the holidays? Do you feel worse around the holidays like Christmas after you've had your fill of luscious chocolates or consumed the food preservatives and colorings often found in fancy holiday cakes and goodies? Or are you worse on birthdays after consuming birthday cake (stirring up wheat/egg allergy) heaped with ice cream (setting off milk allergy)? Since we usually crave the foods to which we're allergic (as well as those we need), it's important to jot down any food that you find yourself craving. Always remember to provide specific details, because they are going to play a major role in tracking down the cause of your allergy. Health care providers can't diagnose evidence that they don't have, so be sure that you record not only every stick of gum, but any spice, seasoning, vitamin, and beverage that you've taken in. If you ate a tuna sandwich for lunch on Friday, don't just write down that you ate tuna salad. Write: tuna, packed in water, with celery and mayonnaise, two slices of white bread, and so on. Record any strange sensations you may have experienced during this time period, no matter how minor it may seem at the time. Bring the diary with you to your health care provider.

Diagnosis

The diagnosis of food allergy generally requires a medical history, physical examination, and diagnostic tests—direct skin tests, blood tests—to rule out other possibilities. In the doctor's office you will have to answer extensive questions about your past and present medical history in order to determine the cause of the allergy. What are the symptoms? Does it include cravings for a certain food? When did the onset of symptoms occur? What types of symptoms do you experience? In addition, you will be asked if you have a history of eczema, asthma, or hay fever, and you will be questioned about your family history of food allergies.

Be sure to thoroughly discuss what diagnostic and treatment plans are anticipated and what they will cost. Always inquire about whether or not allergy tests have been proven effective by accepted standards of scientific evaluation and whether they are FDA approved. Allergies are a hard thing to pinpoint in adults, especially since you may have a negative reaction to food that is not allergic—for example, if you have digestive problems, ulcers, or other medical disorders. With many food allergies, reactions are delayed and consequently hard to trace. If you consume an offending food and develop symptoms hours later, you are unlikely to link your symptoms to the correct substance. An infant, on the other hand, will suffer from distinct and pronounced symptoms and quickly develop a reaction to an allergen. However, an infant may develop an allergic reaction to milk several months after birth. The baby will cry, lose weight, and develop bloody diarrhea. In some adults, symptoms may not show up for several years after exposure to an allergen. An adult may be allergic to a kitten but not develop symptoms until the kitten has grown into a cat.

There has been a great deal of controversy among experts and health care providers over the accuracy of many tests given to diagnose allergy. Some experts assert that one test is most accurate, and others prefer another. The best way to find out which test is right for you is to ask your physician for information about the advantages and drawbacks of each test. Here are some common methods of allergy testing:

Skin Testing The "scratch test" is one of the commonly used forms of skin testing: the outer layers of skin are pierced, and minute amounts of the suspected allergens are placed within the surface break, where antibodies can react to them.

Elimination Diet Both traditional and alternative practitioners use this diet to detect offending food allergens. There are many different forms of the elimination diet, but the general concept is pretty much the same. You begin by excluding a suspected offending food or group of foods from your diet for about a week. During this period, you will be advised to eat foods that are not known to commonly cause allergic reactions. After a week passes, you reintroduce the suspect food or foods; if you develop symptoms when the food is introduced, you know which foods are causing you trouble. If you would like to go on the elimination diet, you must eat the suspected allergenic food before starting the diet so that your body will be exposed to the foods before they are withdrawn. The trial elimination period is about seven days, during which time you will have to ban the suspected offenders from your diet. Not one crumb of a suspected offender should pass between your lips during this seven-day period. Instead you might include rice, appropriate meats, vegetables, fruits, and other foods that are not known to cause allergies. When the week has finished you will slowly reintroduce one food at a time back into your diet. The reintroduced food must be in its purest form—not mixed with other ingredients. That is, if you are testing for milk allergies, you drink a glass of milk. If you are testing for wheat allergies, you fix yourself a bowl of cream of wheat without milk or sugar. If you don't experience a reaction right away, eat the food in its pure form the next time that food is served. Continue to eat the food throughout the day, or until symptoms develop. If you are not experiencing symptoms by bedtime, you can assume that you are not sensitive to that food. Keep the food out of your diet until you have finished testing the other suspected food allergens. If you do happen to react to a food that you are testing, wait until the reaction subsides (about twenty-four to forty-eight hours) before reintroducing the next test food into your diet.

You should never go on an elimination diet without your health care provider's close supervision; and if you get sick—for instance, with the flu—during the diet, you must stop, take care of your illness, and then start over when you're feeling better. Try to plan the diet during a quiet period of the year, when there are no holidays, vacation periods, or family events such as weddings and get-togethers. You may suffer withdrawal symptoms during the initial phase, because your body has to adjust to the absence of foods to which it may have become addicted. Expect these withdrawal symptoms and give your body time to rebound.

Offending Food Once you have been diagnosed with a food allergy, you will be advised to eliminate the offending food from your diet. This is sometimes easier said than done. You will be required to become a food detective, since the content of so many foods can be deceiving. For example, did you know that Hebrew National Hot Dogs now contain wheat? Or that semisweet chocolate is often manufactured on the same assembly line as and thus mixes with other products that contain milk and therefore is not considered a safe food for the milk-allergic individual? When dining out, always ask for the ingredients of any dish you are planning to order. Do you realize that many Chinese restaurants use peanut oil or peanut butter to flavor certain foods? That's important to know if you're allergic to peanuts. Meatballs can be made with everything from eggs to bread crumbs. Hidden sources of milk include chowders, cookies, soup mixtures, gravies, hamburgers, and mashed potatoes. Products that contain wheat can be equally deceptive. If you have a wheat allergy, avoid the following: beer, bran flakes, cornflakes, doughnuts, gin, corn, gluten, lima and graham flour, and malted milk. Eggs, too, come in many disguises, such as macaroons, macaroni, meatballs, sausages, soups, and tartar sauce. Be careful!

Nutritional Substitutes   If you're allergic to certain foods, you may think that cooking will never be the same again. But you can still make your favorite dishes by using these helpful tips, substituting ingredients for the foods that offend your body.

Egg Substitutes

- For binding cakes and pancakes, substitute one banana for one egg.
- For cooking or binding liquids, substitute two tablespoons of cornstarch or arrowroot starch for one egg or substitute two tablespoons of tofu mixed with liquids, until liquefied.

- Substitute Ener-G Egg replacer or similar product for recipes that call for eggs.
- When baking egg-free cookies, lightly grease the cookie sheet to prevent spreading during baking.
- When baking an egg-free cake, slightly increase the amount of ingredients such as raisins, nuts, or spices, to add flavor and texture.
- If a recipe is egg-free or milk-free, it should be baked longer and at a lower heat than the same recipe baked with eggs or milk.

Dairy Replacements

- Use soy milk (available in health food and Asian food stores), soy margarine, and soy yogurt.
- To make nut milks, blend nuts with water and strain.
- To make rice milk, blend cooked rice with water. However, don't use this for baking; use soy milk instead.
- One cup of water or juice mixed with one tablespoon of oil or shortening will serve as a good substitute for one cup of milk.
- Substitute chicken stock for milk in cream soups and casserole recipes.

Epinephrine   If, in spite of all precautions, a food allergen is introduced into the system and results in a severe allergic reaction such as anaphylactic shock, get yourself to an emergency room as quickly as possible. If you have a prior history of anaphylaxis, you should speak to a health care provider about how to self-administer epinephrine. Injectable epinephrine is a synthetic version of a naturally occurring hormone known as adrenaline. In the case of an anaphylactic reaction, a doctor injects it directly in the thigh or vein. It saves lives by reversing throat swelling and allowing you to swallow, relaxing lung muscles to improve breathing, and stimulating the heartbeat among other effects. For emergency home use, epinephrine is available in two forms: a traditional needle-and-syringe kit called Ana-Kit, which contains two doses; or an automatic injector system known as Epi-Pen (with a mechanism that injects the drug automatically) that contains one dose. A physician is best qualified to determine which injectable form should be used by the patient. It is also a good idea to always carry an emergency-care card that lists the foods to which you are allergic, as well as emergency medical contacts and numbers.

Always go to a hospital after an allergic reaction. Mild symptoms can be followed by severe problems within ten to sixty minutes. This holds true whether or not you have injected epinephrine into your system. Although epinephrine may reduce symptoms, you will still require medical observation.

Alternative Treatments   Among the alternative treatments that are available, you will discover different kinds of relief—all natural, but not all suited for your particular condition. Some alternative therapies will fit you like a glove, while others may interfere with allopathic treatments that you are already receiving. You also need to consider what treatment feels right for you. Many health care providers have alleged that they have seen patients eliminate allergy symptoms simply by believing that they had found the cure. If you do not believe in a specific alternative treatment or if it feels uncomfortable in some way, your mind will not allow it to work. Avoid those treatments.

The NIH Office of Alternative Medicine recommends

that people take the following steps before getting involved in alternative therapy:

- Obtain objective information about the therapy. Besides talking with the person promoting the approach, speak with people who have experienced the treatment—preferably both those who were treated recently and those treated in the past. Ask about the advantages and disadvantages, risks, side effects, costs, results, and length of time needed to get results.
- Consider the costs. Alternative treatments are not always reimbursed by health insurance.
- Discuss all treatments with your primary health care provider, who needs this information in order to have a complete picture of your treatment plan.

You must always feel comfortable and confident with any process that is part of your treatment program. If, in addition to being therapeutic, it appeals to your senses and feels wonderful, so much the better.

Testing for Food Allergies

We've already discussed the allopathic method of testing. Food allergy testing in the alternative health field has been touched by controversy. Many of the tests have been dismissed by allopathic practitioners as inaccurate and ineffective. However, advocates of these tests insist that they are valid and do have merit, and they point to case after case of positive results. When it comes to deciding on what tests to have done, the final decision is up to you.

Here are some common tests given by alternative health care providers to detect food allergies:

Food Cytotoxic Blood Test   The food cytotoxic blood test consists of taking a test tube of blood from the patient and mixing the white cells with plasma and water. The mixture is then placed on microscopic slides coated with dried extracts of a particular food. The cells are examined to observe if they have changed shape, disintegrated, or collapsed. Although these tests are given by many alternative health care providers, the FDA does not consider them to be supported by well-controlled studies and clinical trials.

The Pulse Test   In the self-administered pulse test, which should only be given in a quiet and relaxed environment, the pulse is taken after ingestion of a suspected food allergen. Patients take their own pulse before eating the potentially offensive food, and take it again at frequent intervals—at ten, twenty, forty, and sixty minutes—after eating the food. If the pulse rate increases or decreases by more than ten beats per minute, the food is suspect and should be omitted from the diet for one month. At that time testing should be repeated.

Muscle Response Testing   A new method, muscle response testing for allergies is generating a lot of excitement in the field of alternative medicine. A muscle in your body is isolated and exposed to tiny amounts of more than one hundred fifty different allergens, one at a time. Amazingly, every time you come into contact with an allergen, your muscle weakens. Once you discover what you are allergic to, you may begin therapeutic treatment, consisting of carefully integrated acupressure, acupuncture, and non-forceful chiropractic techniques.

Functional Liver Detoxification Profile   A functional liver detoxification profile helps measure the liver's detoxification abilities. A dysfunctional liver can lead to toxicity and a depressed immune system. A chronically impaired liver function can also result in allergic disorders, due to toxicity and lowered immune resistance. The test involves ingesting a small amount of a premeasured caffeine, aspirin, and acetaminophen, then collecting urine and saliva samples one to eight hours later.

Intestinal Permeability Test   The intestinal permeability test is often used where there is suspicion that a malabsorption of food is taking place, as in the case of leaky gut syndrome discussed earlier in this chapter. The test involves the examination of two urine samples, one collected after an overnight fast and the second collected after drinking a premeasured liquid containing two non-metabolized sugar molecules.

Bacterial Overgrowth Breath Test   Bacterial overgrowth often leads to intolerance of dietary carbohydrates, malabsorption, and lowered immune function. Given when allergies are not considered the sole factor contributing to symptoms, the bacterial overgrowth breath test involves the simple and painless process of collecting several breath samples over a period of one and a quarter hours.

Hydrochloric Acid Test   Tests for too little or too much hydrochloric acid in the stomach may be run, since either extreme can be a factor in food allergy.

Dietary Changes

Rotation Diet   Since many food allergies arise because of a repetitive diet, many alternative health care providers will suggest a rotary diet for their patients with allergies. First developed in the 1930s by an allergist named Herbert Rinkel, M.D., the rotary diet is based on the principle that it usually takes four days for a food to "clear" the body. If a food is eaten only once and not repeated for another four days, the body has time to clear itself of antibodies that might create allergy symptoms. The rotary diet allows you to eat small portions of foods that you may be allergic to, and it prevents new allergies from developing due to overexposure.

In order to ensure that your rotary diet is successful, you should take about a week to clear your body of previous allergens by excluding all foods that may have contributed to your symptoms. Once you begin your diet, a different group of foods is eaten once in four days and then the cycle is repeated. The selection of foods for each particular day is up to you or your health care provider. However, it is essential not to eat any food more than once in four days.

The goal of the rotation diet is to keep your food allergy symptoms to a minimum by lessening exposure to known allergens and preventing new allergies from developing. It is recommended that for a period of thirty days you eliminate foods that you are sensitive to and have eaten four or more times a week; then they can be reintroduced into your diet. Don't forget to rotate your beverages, cooking oils, garnishes, and other dietary additions. You might want to keep a notebook to help you remember what you ate and when.

The rotary diet is not a trend or a fad; it's been around for over sixty years because of its success in treating allergies. Common sense dictates that eating too much of one food isn't healthy, and this diet ensures that you diversify your diet and eat a wide variety of foods. Try it. You'll like it.

Vegetarian Diet   Vegetarian diets are often recommended for people with food allergies because they are generally lower in the types of foods that cause allergic reactions. A diet filled with fruits and vegetables tends to include more fresh and unprocessed foods and these are less likely to contain potential preservative, chemical, and food allergens.

What is the best vegetarian diet for you? Ask a nutritionist. A nutritionist will work with you to develop a diet filled with the proper nutrients and vitamins to match your lifestyle, body type, and environmental requirements.

There are three types of vegetarian diets. Strict vegetarian diets eliminate eggs and dairy as well as all meat. Lacto-vegetarian diets permit dairy products. Ovo-lacto-vegetarian diets permit the use of eggs as well as dairy products.

The following suggestions are basic guidelines for keeping a vegetarian diet:

- Save sweets and fatty foods for special occasions.
- Opt for whole, or unrefined, grain products in place of refined flour products whenever possible.
- Eat a variety of fruits and vegetables daily. Introduce new fruits and vegetables into your diet as the source of possible new staples. Dark green vegetables are an especially good source of iron. You can increase your iron absorption by eating foods containing vitamin C along with foods containing iron.
- Use low-fat or nonfat dairy products whenever possible for adult consumption. Children and infants should use regular whole milk, unless otherwise advised.
- Limit your egg intake to three or four yolks per week.
- Vegetarians need a reliable source of vitamin B-12. Good sources are fortified commercial breakfast cereals and fortified soy beverages.
- Use oils, margarine, nuts, nut butters, avocados, and coconut sparingly. They are high in fat. Subscribe to magazines and newsletters that cater to vegetarians. They usually provide good tips for maintaining health and include recipes for variety in your diet. The Vegetarian Resource Group, located in Baltimore, Maryland, puts out an informative bimonthly report.

Herbal Treatments

Sipping a cup of hot tea is a wonderful way to unwind. Commercially prepared herbal teas have other benefits as well. They are an excellent way to soothe the indigestion and stomach upset that often accompany food allergies. Think about it. Wouldn't you rather sip a soothing cup of aromatic peppermint tea instead of gulping down a spoonful of some remedy for indigestion? Isn't the thought of a cup of warm ginger tea infinitely more pleasing than the hard, chalky, taste of an antacid tablet? It isn't hard to get hooked on herbal teas. Many people stock a few brands in their kitchen cabinet and eventually develop strong personal preferences.

Strengths of herbal teas vary according to the individual brand, so check the box to see exactly what you are getting. Generally, the brands that you find in supermarkets are much less potent and more processed than the brands sold in health food stores, and you should keep certain cautions in mind when purchasing your herbal products. A primary health care provider should always be consulted before any herb is used, particularly in the case of pregnant women, children, and people who have certain medical conditions or are using any medication. Do not use any herb for a prolonged period of time, combine herbs on your own, or use any herb in large doses. Some herbs can be toxic even in small doses, so never take a herb you are unfamiliar with or know little about. Be alert for any adverse reactions or side effects, which you should immediately discuss with your primary health care provider.

A good herbal tea to keep in your home is chamomile. You might want to sip a cup of calming chamomile tea (commercially prepared loose tea or teabags steeped ten to fifteen minutes) to remedy the upset stomachs that often accompany food allergies. If you don't care for chamomile, try peppermint! Peppermint and spearmint teas have pleasing aromas and are also noted for their soothing effects. Ginger tea is a classic remedy for digestive problems because it has a healing effect on the digestive system. Once you have decided which teas you prefer, why not add a few tea bags to the company medicine chest, as you would add antacids or aspirin?

Alternative Practitioners

Alternative Health Care Provider   Most alternative health care providers view food allergies as originating in a variety of sources: heredity, a faulty immune system, or even a leaky gut may contribute to allergy symptoms. Alternative health care providers will often treat allergies with the rotary diet discussed earlier in this chapter. If a weakened immune system is considered a factor, nutritional supplements will then be prescribed. If there is a problem with increased intestinal permeability (leaky gut syndrome), your alternative health care provider may prescribe such supplements as amino acids, digestive enzymes, vitamin E, zinc, magnesium, and ascorbic acid, among other supplements. In addition, the alternative practitioner will recommend detoxifying treatments such as gargling apple cider vinegar—one to two teaspoons in a glass of warm water—and plenty of water to flush out toxins. It is important to keep the body clean because a body cleansed with water is less likely to become toxic and more likely to heal faster. To put it simply, a clean body is a healthy body. Drink your water!

Homeopathy   Homeopathic practitioners treat food allergies by prescribing homeopathic solutions that mimic the allergic symptoms for the purpose of eliminating digestive toxins and restoring the body's natural balance. Homeopathic practitioners will initially recommend that you treat the allergy by removing the foods that are causing your symptoms, thus providing relief from your symptoms and boosting the body's healing process.

Many people like the idea of receiving the individualized treatment that homeopathy offers. There is something instinctively tranquilizing about taking remedies from natural substances according to specifications tailored uniquely to your needs. Many traditional allopathic health care providers also have expertise in homeopathy, and the combination of knowledge is excellent when you are seeking advice about homeopathic products. Homeopathic remedies do not, as a rule, interfere with the allopathic allergy medications recommended by your traditional health care provider, so they are a good choice for an integrated program of treatment. For more information about using homeopathic remedies, refer to chapter 2 on adult asthma.

Chiropractor/Nutritionist   Chiropractors who also provide nutritional support can be a strong ally in the war against allergies. Chiropractic adjustments keep your body tuned and functioning to its optimum capacity, which is vitally important when combating an allergic condition. This is not to imply that chiropractic care can cure allergies, because it cannot, but a chiropractor/nutritionist can design a total treatment plan using an array of sophisticated alternative testing methods to uncover "hidden" allergies. With the proper treatment, patients often see rapid results, even after years of neglect and abuse.

A perfect example of the effectiveness of this type of treatment is seen in the story of Carol, who was experiencing severe joint aches and pains, swelling of her hands and feet, and chronic fatigue. She had also begun to look rather unhealthy, with dark circles under her eyes and a pale, listless complexion. Her problem was finally resolved when, in addition to her chiropractic treatments, she was given a battery of tests to uncover the cause of her condition. Though physical examination was unremarkable, and her comprehensive digestive stool analysis was within normal limits, her intestinal permeability test revealed that she was suffering from leaky gut syndrome. In addition, her seven-day history revealed that Carol ate the same foods every day and that her protein intake was woefully inadequate. The only protein that she took in was a tiny amount of tuna and eggs. The balance of her diet consisted of bread, rice, and pasta. She also drank an average of twenty-four ounces of citrus juice every day. When allergy tests were run, they revealed that she was allergic to citrus, eggs, rye, oats, and a few environmental allergens. Carol had a classic craving for all of the foods that she was allergic to and/or perhaps addicted to. Carol was put on a rotary diet and given supplements such as L. Glutamine and Prodophilus Complex to normalize her leaky gut. And she was told to increase her water intake to eighty ounces a day and to take vitamin C supplements, along with 500 mgs of Pantothenic acid, 2000 mgs of Glucosamine Sulfate, and a mix of antioxidants daily. Her complexion is no longer listless, and her dark circles are now completely gone, driving home the point that you can't look good if you're not healthy.

TREATMENTS FOR FOOD ALLERGIES

Conventional	Alternative
Diet	*Diet*
Avoidance of food allergens	Rotary, vegetarian, elimination
Journal	*Journal*
Diary to link symptoms with foods	Diary to track foods during rotary diet
Antacids	*Herbal Treatments*
	Homeopathy
	Custom remedies

Combined Treatments

When it comes to treating food allergies, the solution is relatively simple: Identify the offending food or foods and eliminate it/them from your diet. Addressing additional factors, such as repairing the immune system and ridding the body of mucus and toxins, can be achieved through a variety of steps described throughout this chapter. An allopathic health care provider can assist in the healing process by offering consultation and testing to help you pinpoint the cause of your allergies, and even perhaps save your life with wonder drugs such as epinephrine in the case of an anaphylactic reaction. An alternative health care provider can, first, supplement your initial treatment plan with bodywork techniques to free your body of the stress and tension that may aggravate allergies, and, second, offer options such as herbal teas and recipes, which you can alternate with antacids and nonprescription remedies to avoid harmful side effects and chemical dependence. Some of the allopathic and natural treatment options can be combined to suit your specific needs.

Once you have been properly diagnosed and have pinpointed the allergy, you may want to discuss the following natural supplements with your primary health care provider:

- Keep your colon healthy with acidophilus cultures—eat lots of yogurt—particularly if you have recently been given a course of antibiotics. Include fiber in your diet to keep your colon clean. Consult a nutritionist if necessary. Try not to overuse antacids—which brings us to our next tip!
- Use herbal treatments to complement your allopathic treatment program. Substitute a cup of commercially prepared chamomile, peppermint tea, or slippery elm tablets for your usual antacid.
- Consider adopting a strict vegetarian diet or perhaps just simply adding more vegetables and fruits; also consider eliminating many of the processed foods in your diet. Very few people can claim to be allergic to spinach and brussels sprouts, although some may wish they were.
- Learn how to use the rotation diet to avoid developing new allergies. Preventing allergies is just as important as treating them. Treat with medication, heal with food!

CHAPTER 7

Food Sensitivities

Your symptoms include bloating, diarrhea, gas, cramps, and irritability. You love milk, but it doesn't seem to love you back. You lust after grilled cheese sandwiches, cheese and crackers, and cones heaped with rich chocolate ice-cream. But shortly after eating these foods you feel gassy and cramped and desperately sorry that you even thought about the word dairy. If this scenario sounds familiar, you might be suffering from what is classified as a food sensitivity.

FOOD INTOLERANCE

A food sensitivity is not an allergy, although it may feel like one. Unlike an allergy, it does not involve the body's immune system. Rather, it is a metabolic problem, and it is much more common than food allergy.

There are various forms of food sensitivity, and one of the most common is undoubtedly lactose intolerance, which is so widespread simply because milk products are so common in the typical American diet. Without the lactase enzyme, which lactose-intolerant people lack, the intestine cannot break down lactose into glucose and galactose. In addition, several conditions—including infectious diarrhea, intestinal parasites, and inflammatory bowel disease—damage the intestinal lining and lead to lactose malabsorption. Certain individuals, among them alcoholics, people suffering from malnutrition, or those who have taken heavy doses of antibiotics, are more vulnerable to developing problems with lactose malabsorption. You won't find many milk products in Japan, but it is interesting to note that Asians and people of African ancestry suffer from the highest level of lactose deficiency, while northern Europeans suffer the least.

Other kinds of food intolerance include:

Fructose Intolerance

Fructose is used as a sweetener in many soft drinks and is present in certain fruits. The symptoms of intolerance to fructose are similar to those of lactose intolerance.

Sucrose Intolerance

Kiss your sweet tooth good-bye! People who suffer from sucrose intolerance are sensitive to common table sugar. The sucrase enzyme is needed to break down sucrose into glucose and fructose. If you test negative for lactose intolerance but continue to experience symptoms of food sensitivity, you might want to be tested for sucrose intolerance.

Maltose Intolerance

If you suffer from maltose intolerance, you cannot tolerate the maltase enzyme needed for breakdown of maltose into two molecules of glucose.

Additives

Refer to chapter 6 on food allergies for a list of additives and the symptoms that they produce. Some of the additives are classified as food allergens, while others are not but produce symptoms of food sensitivity among some individuals.

Other causes of food sensitivities

Some people may experience temporary symptoms of food sensitivity at times when they are angry, sad, or experiencing other strong emotions. Sometimes serious disorders, even cancer, can be the cause of allergylike symptoms that mimic food sensitivity. The only way to discover exactly what is causing your symptoms is to consult with your health care provider.

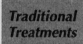
Traditional Treatments

The bad news is that you are suffering from a food sensitivity. The good news is that you have discovered that it is not a food allergy as you had first assumed. That's half of the battle. Many people put off seeing a health care provider because they feel that they can simply take an antacid tablet and they will be OK. The truth is that they are simply masking symptoms that eventually will have to be addressed. Food sensitivity is not a benign condition: chronic sensitivities, such as lactose intolerance, can lead to other medical conditions—for example, an overgrowth of bacteria and yeast, malabsorption, increased susceptibility to infection, and systemic symptoms such as low immunity and hormonal imbalance. Any time that our bodies have trouble handling a food that is consumed, complications can and will set in.

Diagnosis

It is always best to see a health care provider if you suspect food sensitivities because suspicion alone is not enough of a reason to eliminate a food from your diet. There are different degrees of sensitivity to specific foods, and small amounts of a food to which you are sensitive may still be included in your diet. You might also be suffering from a medical disorder that produces similar symptoms, such as ulcers, diarrhea, irritable bowel syndrome; there are also other serious conditions that require specific medical attention and care. This is why proper testing and diagnosis are very important.

Adjusting Your Diet

One of the primary ways to test for lactose intolerance is simply by eliminating all milk products from the diet. However, this is not always the most effective option because many foods and drugs have lactose as a filler, making it nearly impossible to totally eliminate milk products from the diet. In addition, it is not wise to completely remove milk from the diet of certain individuals, especially pregnant and lactating women, infants, and growing children.

One way of determining whether you are sensitive to certain foods is by keeping a diary of what foods you ate during the day, when symptoms developed, and the specific kinds of symptoms that developed. This is a vital record to bring to your primary health care provider to assist in the diagnosis of your condition. In addition to perusing your diary, the health care provider will take your medical history and run tests for food allergies in order to rule out that possibility.

If it is determined that you are indeed suffering from lactose, sucrose, maltose, or fructose intolerance, you will be asked to eliminate certain foods containing those enzymes from your diet. In the case of lactose intolerance, total elimination may not always be necessary because you may be able to add lactase enzyme preparations to milk products to help you digest them. If you suffer from lactose intolerance, chances are you avoid dairy products. If this is the case, you need to obtain calcium from other sources. Foods that are rich in calcium are kelp, chick-peas, broccoli, cabbage, parsley, carrots, summer squash, onions, salmon, sardines, shrimp, clams, cod, oysters, grains and nuts, pistachios, sesame seeds, soy milk, oat flakes, buckwheat, cream of wheat, whole wheat, brown rice, figs, maple syrup, and eggs. Blackstrap molasses has more calcium than milk.

To replace milk when cooking and baking you can use soy milk, soy margarine, soy yogurt, nut milks, or rice milk which should be used for cooking only since it doesn't bake well. Refer to chapter 6 on food allergies for more information on nutritional substitutes.

Just because a food says "nondairy" does not mean that it is free from milk derivatives. Coffee whiteners, for example, contain a milk derivative called caseinate. Under a new FDA ruling, caseinate will have to be identified as a milk derivative in the list of ingredients given on foods that claim to be non-dairy. Here is a list of other "hidden sources" of lactose:

- chocolate
- cocoa drinks
- hot dogs, luncheon meats, sausage
- mashed potatoes
- mayonnaise and salad dressing made with milk
- nondairy creamers (except for Coffee Rich)
- prepared flour mixes (cake, cookies, muffins, pancakes)
- sherbets
- soups
- tuna

- prescription medicines including birth control pills
- many vitamins
- anything labeled whey, casein, lactalbumin and lactose

Nonprescription medications

Many people who suffer from food sensitivities may on occasion consume a "hidden source" of the food that they are sensitive to. In that case, many rely on a traditional form of relief in the guise of stomach powders, solutions, and tablets such as Tums and Mylanta that neutralize or counteract acidity. You may use these products occasionally, but they should not become part of your usual routine. If you find that you need to use these remedies on a regular basis, you should discuss this problem with your physician.

In addition to the regular class of antacids a new group of products for gastric relief have hopped from the pharmacist's counter to the drugstore shelves. Tagamet, Zantac, and Pepcid, previously obtained only by prescription, are now readily available over the counter for treating heartburn and acid indigestion. They differ from the usual antacids that immediately neutralize any acid that's present, since these H2 blockers must enter the bloodstream before they can begin to work, which means they take as long as fifteen to thirty minutes to give relief. The advantage to taking these medications, even though they are slow to start, is that they slow the production of stomach acid and provide relief for up to twelve hours, much longer than regular antacids. The medications that are available in nonprescription form are weaker in dosage than those that are available by prescription. However, that doesn't mean that they aren't effective. Tagamet, Zantac, and Pepcid are all very safe and quite effective for treating occasional heartburn and providing gastric relief. To be on the safe side, however, there are certain precautions that you should take when using any of these medications. You should contact your doctor if you experience vomiting, unexplained weight loss, difficulty swallowing, pain, or evidence of internal bleeding such as black stools. Tagamet HB may interact negatively with other drugs. And you should consult your physician before taking theophylline, often prescribed for asthma, emphysema, or chronic bronchitis; warfin, a blood thinner; or phenytoin, a seizure medication.

Alternative Treatments The alternative medical world has always put a heavy emphasis on the role of food and nutrition in maintaining the health of the body. It may be for this reason that alternative health care providers have excelled in developing tests and treatments for food allergies and food sensitivities. In this section you will discover the latest alternative testing methods, as well as therapies for the safe and effective relief of symptoms through time-tested remedies.

Breath Hydrogen/Methane Testing

The breath hydrogen/methane test has become the standard for testing lactose intolerance as well as intolerance to carbohydrates such as fructose (fruit sugar), sucrose (table sugar), and maltose. The Great Smokies Laboratory in North Carolina, which offers this noninvasive assessment of lactase deficiency, cites several reasons why their breath test for lactose intolerance offers several advantages over other testing. One advantage is the test's greater specificity in determining the degree of malabsorption, which helps health care providers tailor their treatment plans to the individual patient's precise requirements. For example, a person who has been tested and shown only mild absorption problems may simply have to reduce lactose intake by cutting milk consumption in half. By making this change, the patient can eliminate symptoms and still enjoy some milk products. It is also important to remember that not every milk product contains great amounts of lactose. Milk contains a great deal of lactose and may create problems, while cream cheese contains very little and may not produce any symptoms in some individuals. Lactose-sensitive patients may also reduce their lactose intake by using products such as Lactaid, a lactose-reduced milk. Eating a solid (nondairy) food while drinking a glass of milk can also increase tolerance. For those whose tests have shown more severe absorption problems, using lactase enzyme and other commercial preparations has been shown to be helpful.

How is the breath hydrogen/methane test given? Generally, the patient is asked to fast overnight and then to collect a breath sample for testing. Technological advances have made breath testing a relatively simple process, and breath samples can be taken at home or in the health care provider's office. Samples are collected using a breath test kit, which makes use of a simple mouthpiece (patent pending), and vacuum-sealed tubes. By means of the mouthpiece, patients blow into the vacuum-sealed tubes, which puncture the self-sealing mechanism, allowing a breath sample to be collected in the tube for testing. After samples are collected at one-, two-, and three-hour intervals, they are examined to see if the lactose has been broken down. If the lactose has not been broken down by the lactase enzyme in the small intestine, it will travel to the colon where it will undergo bacterial fermentation. Because of this fermentation, hydrogen methane levels in the breath will rise in one to two hours. Test results determine whether there is a lactase deficiency and the degree of intolerance.

Alternative Health Care Provider

An alternative health care provider assesses food sensitivities by asking a variety of questions. What do you eat? When do you eat it? Is your lifestyle stressful or calm? What are your symptoms and how long have you had them? Are you breaking out in rashes? Is your body rebelling with symptoms such as bloating and diarrhea? Are you listening to your body or simply ignoring the symptoms? Natural medicine treats the cause of the problem as well as the symptoms. Although you will be given treatments to relieve your symptoms, you will be asked to eliminate any food from your diet to which you are found to be sensitive. After methods such as the elimination diet (see chapter 6 on food allergies) have uncovered the cause of your sensitivity, a diet will be designed to rid your body of toxins, to provide adequate and alternative nourishment, and coax your system back to good health. Most important, you will be treated as a unique individual, and the particular factors affecting your specific sensitivities will be considered in designing your treatment plan. Possible treatments might include acupressure for strengthening the immune system, homeopathy to relieve gastrointestinal symptoms, and herbal medicine, and/or hydrotherapy to detoxify the digestive system.

Acupressure

We digest our food best when we are relaxed and our bodies are functioning properly. Acupressure—much like its predecessor acupuncture—was designed to correct systemic imbalances, as in the digestive system. The appeal of these techniques lies in hands-on contact and their lack of toxic ingredients, which make them an ideal complement to chemical medications in digestive problems. Although acupressure is beneficial, however, it is not meant to substitute for medical care and should be used only as part of a total treatment program.

Two techniques are designed specifically for self-application. One, called *Acu-yoga*, makes use of whole body postures along with deep breathing, finger pressure, meditation techniques, and stretches. *Do-in* also incorporates body awareness, stretching, and breathing techniques, but is much more energetic and vigorous in its approach. Its focus is on stimulating the points and meridians of the body.

Whether you try it yourself or get a professional acupressure massage, you will find acupressure most helpful in enhancing digestion. Always discuss your digestive problems and overall health with your acupressure practitioner before you begin treatment.

Herbal Treatments

Commercially prepared herb remedies are the natural alternative to pharmaceuticals in relieving stomach upset, nausea, gas, and bloating. They are inexpensive and easy to use, and a little bit of herb goes a long way in relieving symptoms of food sensitivity. Again, before you start experimenting with herbs you should always consult your primary health care provider, particularly in the case of pregnant women, children, and people who have a medical condition or are using any medication. Do not use any herb for a prolonged period of time, combine herbs on your own, or use any herb you are unfamiliar with or know little about. Be alert for any adverse reactions or side effects, which you should immediately discuss with your primary health care provider.

Here are some herbs that can be useful in treating food sensitivity:

Peppermint Tea   Peppermint tea smells delightful, lifts the spirits, and relieves such symptoms as indigestion and nausea. Its pleasant aroma and taste make it a wonderful substitute for store-bought antacids. It can be purchased loose or in tea bags at the health food store.

Chamomile   The Anglo-Saxons looked upon chamomile as one of the nine sacred herbs given to mankind by the god Woden to heal the world. It is indeed a wonderful herb, especially when its strongly scented flowers are used as a tea for soothing digestion. It is sold loose or in tea bags at supermarkets and health food stores.

Ginger   A classic remedy for an upset stomach, ginger can be purchased in capsules, crystallized candy, or in dried ginger root. You can purchase ginger root tea in the health food store. Steer clear of the overprocessed and sugary brands found in commercial supermarkets.

Slippery Elm   Often used to treat inflammation of the stomach, slippery elm bark tablets are among the best natural solutions to take for stomach upset because they help line the stomach and reduce stomach inflammation. Take one to two 200-gram capsules to treat indigestion, gastritis, and stomach upset.

Golden Seal   Golden Seal is used in cases of food sensitivity to promote improved digestion and liver function. Do not use it, however, if you have high blood pressure or if you are pregnant.

Meadowsweet   An excellent remedy for gastritis and stomach upsets, meadowsweet can be used in the form of a tincture to treat stomach symptoms stemming from food sensitivities. This is another treatment that should be avoided by children and pregnant women.

Diet and Nutrition

During the course of treatment for food sensitivity by an alternative health care practitioner, your diet will have to be fine-tuned to your individual requirements. Once food sensitivity is established, measures will be taken to alter the diet and correct any problems that have been caused by food intolerance and malabsorption. The following diet and nutritional measures can be taken:

- *Remove all milk products from your diet.* This includes all "hidden sources" of lactose, including bread and baked goods, salad dressings, and other foods containing milk.
- *Identify and correct any nutrient deficiencies.* Serious nutritional deficiencies can result from chronic malabsorption problems. Supplement your diet with nutrient-rich foods to remedy vitamin and mineral deficiencies.
- *Administer friendly flora if you discover a deficiency.* Lactobacilli are friendly bacteria that will enhance digestion of lactose by producing the enzyme lactase. They also aid in the absorption and digestion of nutrients. If you wish to be a cordial host or hostess to your friendly bacteria, start by feeding them properly with fermented dairy foods such as yogurt. It is especially important to replenish your supply of friendly bacteria if you have just finished a course of antibiotics, which tend to destroy healthy gut flora. You can also lend them a hand by eating heavy-fiber foods such as bran, sprouts, and carrots to keep the colon clean so that the bacteria will thrive.
- *Adding extra calcium to your diet.* If milk must be removed from the diet, provide substitutes for calcium in the form of foods such as sardines, vegetables, grains, nuts, brown rice, and eggs.

Homeopathic Remedies

Especially in conjunction with a total treatment plan, homeopathic remedies will stimulate your body to heal itself and relieve symptoms of food sensitivity such as diarrhea, nausea, and digestive upset. As discussed previously, homeopathic remedies should be tailored specifically for your unique needs by a homeopathic practitioner. (Refer to the discussion of homeopathic treatment in chapter 2.) The following remedies are commonly prescribed:

- *Arsenicum album* is often used to treat food poisoning that has resulted in diarrhea.
- *Podophyllum* helps relieve diarrhea.
- *Nux vomica* is used to treat gastrointestinal problems such as upset stomach, abdominal bloating, and heartburn.

TREATMENTS FOR FOOD SENSITIVITY

Conventional	Alternative
Diet	*Diet and Nutritional Supplements*
Removal of the offending food from the diet	Bio-Detox, Probiotics, L-Glutamine, L-Gluthathione and other antioxidants, Ultra Clear Sustain, L. bulgaricus
Nonprescription Medications	*Herbal Teas*
Zantac 75, Tagamet HB, Pepcid AC, Antacids, Axid AR	
	Acupressure
	Acu-yoga, Do-in
Lactase supplements	*Homeopathy*
	Custom remedies

Combined Treatments

In the case of food intolerance and sensitivity, avoiding or reducing consumption of the foods that offend you is an essential key to successful treatment. Allopathic or natural testing to identify the offending food or foods is a major part of resolving your problem. Testing is particularly important because food allergies and sensitivities are commonly confused, even though they are distinctly different conditions. Once your condition is clarified, however, a diet can be put into place that will resolve your problem. Another reason why proper testing is so important is that not everyone who is intolerant of a food needs to eliminate it entirely from the diet. Precise testing methods such as the hydrogen/methane test for intolerances to lactose, fructose, sucrose, and maltose can determine the precise degree of intolerance so that a treatment might include some of the foods that may previously have had to be avoided. Work with your primary health care practitioner to design a total treatment plan. Together, you might decide that you should:

- Add homeopathic remedies that are custom designed to your individual needs to boost your body's healing powers.
- Use bodywork therapies such as acupressure to supplement the allopathic medications you are taking to relieve symptoms. Acupressure massage supports your body's recovery, and it can lessen your dependence on nonprescription gastric-relief medications by helping you relax, which aids digestion. Learn acupressure techniques that you can use at home to soothe the symptoms of food sensitivity when they arise.
- Work with your health care provider to ensure you are maintaining healthy gut flora through diet and/or sup-

plements. If food sensitivity has led to malabsorption of nutrients, work with a nutritionist to design a diet of nutrient-dense foods that will nourish your body.

- Alternate use of antacids with natural stomach soothers such as slippery elm tablets or meadowsweet tincture (if you are not pregnant).

CHAPTER 8

Industrial and Environmental Allergies

They are powerful, toxic, and they are everywhere. They are in our offices, homes, food, and our water—in the very air that we breathe. They can make you break out in hives or itch, wheeze, and cough. They could very well be the source behind those constant nagging headaches or the unexplained muscle aches you've been experiencing. They are industrial and inorganic allergens, and you are at their mercy.

We have come a long way with air pollution controls on cars and in our factories. But we also use a lot more chemicals in our homes and our workplaces. We no longer clean our houses with baking soda and vinegar or mild soap. We use fancy detergents and harsh chemicals for cleaning, and our workplaces expose us to poisonous chemicals such as chlorine, fluorine, bromine, or iodine. We sprinkle our lawns with toxic pesticides to protect us from insects and to keep our grass green. But do we realize what it does to our nervous systems?

Pesticides are in our groceries; fumes and dirty air are in our offices; and chemicals are in our food. And our office buildings are now being built with windows designed to stay closed, which means that the fumes don't get out. In place of fresh air, we have poor ventilation systems that impede circulation, forming a dangerous suspension of bacteria, fumes, chemicals, and germs in the atmosphere. Some people don't suffer any symptoms, while others feel sluggish, depressed, and irritated.

In dealing with these allergies it is important to assume nothing. If you experience symptoms, don't diagnose yourself. Consult with your primary health care provider to determine whether the cause of your symptoms is in fact an industrial or inorganic allergy. Different types of allergy require different treatments. The symptoms most often associated with industrial or inorganic allergies include sinus problems, coughing, eczema, hives, vomiting, gas, constipation, diarrhea, depression, and sluggishness. Keep a record of your symptoms—when, where, and how often they appear. This valuable information will help you and your health care provider determine exactly what is causing them.

WHAT CAUSES INDUSTRIAL AND INORGANIC ALLERGIES?

The body is constantly bombarded by a barrage of foreign substances that some people—in particular those with weakened immune systems or poor diets, children, the elderly, the frail—cannot tolerate. Even people with strong immune systems, if they come into contact with highly toxic substances, will begin to suffer symptoms. Some common industrial and inorganic offenders are:

- industrial waste
- pesticides
- gasoline
- dry-cleaning chemicals

- household cleaners
- paint
- perfumes
- disinfectants
- laundry detergents
- alcohol

Chemical substances that are commonly found to be allergens include methyl bromide (found in dried fruits and nuts), petrochemicals, halogens, lead, mercury, asbestos, sulfur, ammonia, fluorine, bromine, iodine, dioxin (a weed killer), and polybrominated biphenyl (a fire retardant). Each day we are exposed to a massive array of environmental pollutants. Radon (for which there are home tests; call the EPA Radon Hotline at (800) SOS-RADON for an information kit), asbestos (insulation found in building materials), and formaldehyde (a colorless, strong-smelling, and potentially cancer-causing gas) are present in our building materials, insulation, and furnishings. We inhale ammonia fumes as we clean our homes with store-bought cleaning products. Potential environmental allergens such as pollen, molds, and spores are all found in close proximity. And, ironically, our drinking water—which is supposed to cleanse and replenish us—is tainted with industrial emissions.

Chemicals are also in our foods. Metasulfites are found in food, wine, and beer as well as in potatoes and shellfish. Sodium benzoate is associated with migraine headaches and tartrazine, also called FD&C Yellow No. 5, is a common ingredient of our snacks and daily meals. Harmful dusts from grain, feathers, mold, and fur can cause allergies in people who work with these substances or are exposed to them regularly.

Who is most susceptible to developing allergic reactions

to chemicals and other inorganic materials? Factors may include, among others, a genetic predisposition to develop allergies, poor nutrition, leaky gut syndrome (see chapter 6), exposure to pesticides and other chemicals, high stress, and frequent use of antibiotics. Individuals at high risk include people who work in energy-sealed buildings or who breathe in fumes from office equipment, chemicals, and other inhalants in the workplace; potters and artists who work with solvents, metal fumes, ink, and clay; factory workers who handle chemicals, detergents, or plastics; people who live in parts of the country with heavy smog and toxins; dry cleaners, hairdressers, printers, and the unborn children of these men and women.

An example of how unpredictably allergies can develop is clearly demonstrated in the case of a vigorous young intern—let's call him William—who worked in the emergency room of a small hospital. After a few years of working there, he developed health problems with symptoms such as fatigue, shortness of breath, tearing eyes, and other classic signs of allergy. But the source of these allergies was a mystery in spite of extensive testing.

A skin test was performed and no allergies were found. A methocol test (which tests lungs sensitivity) also failed to uncover allergies. William thought that he'd overlooked nothing in his search for the cause of his allergies, and he was right—except for one consideration. A year earlier, the hospital had purchased a high-temperature incinerating system that was located near the on-call room. *The hospital itself was making William sick!* William did eventually leave the hospital; however, this story does not have an entirely happy ending. Although his initial allergy was gone, his entire system had, due to the allergy, become highly sensitive to multiple allergy triggers. So, although his original allergy problems did improve, he continues to live with an increased level of sensitivity to allergens in the environment: an allergic reaction to certain pollutants introduces new sensitivities to other irritants, creating a vicious and irreversible cycle. The case of William warns us about the dangers of inorganic pollution in the workplace.

Traditional Treatments If you suspect that you are suffering from environmental allergies, you should visit either a health care provider who is experienced in dealing with inorganic and industrial allergies or, in the case of occupational and industrial allergies, an occupational medical specialist. As yet, there are no reliable tests to diagnose allergic reactions to most chemical toxins. Since there are literally thousands of industrial toxins, the screening process would be far too expensive and extensive for practical purposes. Allergy tests such as the skin test might be able to detect dust allergies, but there's not much you can do about them except to limit your contact to the extent that is possible.

Here are some possible allopathic options for detecting sensitivity, keeping in mind that not all of these are effective:

Physical Examinations

A thorough physical examination will be given by your primary health care provider, along with the taking of a medical, work, lifestyle, and family history. Laboratory tests and X rays also will be taken. You will be asked about the symptoms you are experiencing, their onset, and where—specific locations—they occur. By keeping track of your reactions and symptoms in a diary (see below), you may help to pinpoint possible allergens as well as assist your doctor to rule out other possible causes of your symptoms. Industrial and inorganic allergies are treated like other allergies: first the allergy must be diagnosed; once discovered, its cause must be avoided to whatever extent is possible; and finally, symptoms must be relieved.

Skin Testing

Skin testing is generally performed when an allergic reaction to dust mites, molds, or pollen, food, or chemicals is suspected. The most common form of skin testing is the scratch test, in which the surface of the skin is scratched with a fine needle, a solution is applied, and reactions are observed. Skin tests such as the prick test are also effective in detecting inhalant allergies. See chapter 4 for details.

Journal/Daily Log

When you walk into your doctor's office complaining of chemical allergies, or muscle aches and pains, the doctor will take a thorough medical history and run a battery of tests to determine your overall health. The primary tool used in detecting industrial and inorganic allergies is the diary that you should have been keeping to precisely record your symptoms. This diary should provide the data for the followings questions: When do your symptoms appear? How often? Are they worse at work than they are at home? Do they seem to coincide with activities that you are engaged in at a particular time? Are you exposed to chemicals during the day? Which chemicals? Do the symptoms begin during or after the time that you are in a particular location?

Once the source and type of allergen is identified, there are a number of treatment options to follow:

Immunotherapy (allergy injections)

Immunotherapy could be one solution to your allergies, particularly in the case of such environmental allergens as dust mites and mold allergies. Refer to the discussion of immunotherapy in chapter 2 on adult asthma for more details about this method of treatment.

Avoidance

Avoidance is the first step to take in treating allergies; it is the approach that will initially be recommended by your health care provider. It may be easy to get rid of allergens in some cases, but as we have seen in the case of the intern named William, who was allergic to his workplace, it may not always be possible. If allergies are extremely severe, a change of job or even of occupation may be necessary eventually. If you are having such a problem, speak to your employers about making some changes in your environment. If you think there is a violation of workplace safety regulations, you might want to call your local branch of the Occupational Safety and Health Administration (OSHA) and file a confidential report (the law protects your privacy). If allergies are found predominantly in your home, detergents, household cleaners and pesticides have to be eliminated.

Below are some tips for eliminating or reducing the amount of toxic chemicals and allergens in your home and office.

In the home:

- Use natural pesticides on your lawn and in the garden. Herbal sprays and foods such as chili pepper, mint, thyme, rosemary, and other natural substances naturally repel insects. There are many books available that offer excellent recipes for natural pesticides.

- Use natural household products whenever possible. White vinegar mixed with water makes a great glass cleaner. Baking soda is excellent for fighting mold and odors without having to use chemicals. And mixed with vinegar, baking soda makes a great deodorizing toilet-bowl cleaner. To remove mildew, mix half a cup of vinegar with half a cup of borax and water. If you don't want to prepare your own products, you can purchase natural household cleaning products from your health food store.
- Increase the circulation of air throughout the house.
- Remove all containers of pesticides, mothballs, and fly strips from the house. Stay indoors when your neighbor's lawn is being fertilized or sprayed with toxic chemicals.
- As in the case of the doctor who became sensitive to chemicals after long exposure to an allergen, you may have been left with an increased sensitivity to a number of chemicals. When you are traveling, you might opt to stay in what is known as an EverGreen room. Some hotels and motels in thirteen states have set aside rooms that provide a smoke-free, allergen-free atmosphere as well as filtered drinking water. For more details call EverGreen Room Properties at (800) 929-2626 from 9 A.M. to 5 P.M. EST on weekdays.

In the office:

- Try to avoid working in air-conditioned offices with sealed windows.
- Make sure that the office photocopying machine is in a well-ventilated spot.

- Wear all of the protective clothing provided by your job.
- Avoid solvents. Wear protective masks when using them.
- Surround yourself with plants that absorb pollutants. Plants that do this best include chrysanthemums, devil's ivy, English ivy, orchids, yellow tulips, and the peace lily.
- Request that you be notified of any painting, renovation, or application of cleaning products that emit strong fumes or contain irritants. Try to move to a different office or floor far away from the work area.

Alternative Treatments   Alternative treatments are a particularly suitable way to counteract the assault of chemicals, pollution, and modern technology, as well as the negative energies that are part of the competitive work world. What could be a more appropriate response to chemicals, smog, exhaust, and pesticides than finding such natural remedies as fresh herbs, clean water, and a relaxing massage?

Diagnosis

When you arrive at your alternative health care provider, you will be given a physical examination that will lead to an initial diagnosis. After the initial examination if the practitioner suspects industrial or inorganic allergies, one or more of the following tests will be administered:

Intracutaneous One-to-Five Serial Dilution Titration

In intracutaneous one-to-five serial dilution titration, a small amount of an allergen is inserted into the skin, causing a wheal about the size of a typical mosquito bite to form; if you are allergic, the size of the wheal will increase within ten minutes.

Clinical Titration In the clinical titration, excitants (environmental chemicals) are given intracutaneously—shot in the arm or given as drops under the tongue—to provoke the allergic reaction. The reactions are then measured to determine sensitivity.

Functional Liver Detoxification Profile The liver is a primary player in the body's defense system. It converts and neutralizes toxins into safe by-products, which are then eliminated. When pollutants and toxic chemicals challenge this defense system, the overload can lead to systemic damage that may also result in the development of allergies. A functional liver detoxification profile is usually taken to assess how well the liver is functioning to eliminate toxic chemicals. The test involves the collection of urine and saliva samples after the ingestion of a small premeasured amount of caffeine, aspirin, and acetaminophen.

Various Therapies

Once the cause of your allergies has been determined, a treatment program can be designed to meet your needs. Following are some therapies that may be used to restore your body to good health.

Massage Swedish massage assists the body's healing process by stimulating the release of toxins, increasing circulation of the blood that nourishes body tissues, and reducing muscle aches and fatigue. It also promotes overall general relaxation so that the body can release the stress that may be contributing to your allergies. Scheduling a weekly massage is a good idea as part of a total treatment plan for your allergies. Be sure that you are comfortable with the practitioner and that you have selected a form of massage that you find particularly relaxing. Some people prefer deep massage movements and others prefer a lighter touch. Giving feedback about personal preferences and areas that are particularly tense is important for optimum benefit. Be sure to inform the therapist about your present allergies condition so that he or she can suggest specific massage options. In a seaweed massage, seaweed is applied externally over the skin to reduce toxins; an aromatherapy massage incorporates essential oils and floral water sprays to relieve stress and both stimulate and relax the body.

Herbal Treatments   The natural power of herbs can do much to counteract the damage caused by contact with chemicals and inorganic pollution. Since your body is already extremely sensitive, be very careful about what you put into it. It is important to consult with an herbal practitioner as well as your physician to learn about the appropriate and safe way to use herbs to treat symptoms and cleanse toxins. It is best to use commercially prepared herbal recipes to avoid the danger of toxic effects. As mentioned previously, always consult with your primary health care provider before taking herbal remedies—especially if you are pregnant or are regularly using other medications.

Do not store your herbal preparations in plastic containers: the plastic tends to absorb reactive chemicals that may be present in many herbs. Dark glass bottles are normally used for storing herbal solutions because the dark color protects the mixture from alteration by sunlight and heat. If you have purchased a herb in powdered form and find it less than palatable, you might want to convert the powder into capsule form. Capsules are very convenient and are easy to administer; unfortunately they are not always readily available. If the herb that you wish to purchase does not come in capsule form, you can buy the powdered herb and prepare your own capsules at home. In order to make your own herbal capsules, you will need a saucer or flat dish, some capsule cases (gelatin or vegetarian), and an airtight container for storage. Start by pouring the powdered herb into the saucer or flat dish. Separate the two halves of a capsule case and slide them through the powder, scooping it up. Then fit the two halves of the capsule case together and place in an airtight container.

Milk Thistle Although farmers and the uninitiated view this valuable herb as merely a pesky weed, milk thistle is legendary for protecting, strengthening, and repairing the liver. Lonicern, a fifteenth-century herbalist, was the first to write about its usefulness. Milk thistle has a protective effect against chemicals, which makes it an ideal remedy for treating industrial and inorganic allergies. Although it is generally safe for most people, the elderly, children, and pregnant women should not take it. To prepare it for ingestion, steep one teaspoon of the commercially prepared herb in one cup of boiling water for about fifteen minutes. Drink one to three cups a day. Do not exceed this amount.

Ginseng Ginseng supports the adrenal glands, has a calming effect on the nervous system, and enhances all bodily functions. It is classed as an "adaptogen," which increases the overall resistance of the body to all kinds of stress. Other herbal adaptogens include astragalus, Siberian ginseng, and schizandra. The key to the successful use of ginseng as a tonic, when approved by your primary health care provider, is to take a small amount daily on a regular basis. Using megadoses in spurts to build up vitality is an exercise in futility. You should avoid taking coffee, soya beans, or turnips for at least three hours after using ginseng, since they counteract its effects. One or two grams a day of ginseng is recommended when you experience mental and physical stress, although pregnant women, children, the elderly, and/or those with medical conditions such as high blood pressure or heart problems should first consult their health care provider. There are different grades of ginseng, and the price difference can be substantial. Usually, the ordinary grade will suffice.

Passion Flower The name of this herb hints at stimulation, but passion flower actually has a calming effect and is often used with other sedative herbs to treat nervous conditions. It may be taken as an antidote to the stress of working in a toxic environment.

Lavender The Romans used lavender to scent bath water, and it was regarded by them as an excellent sedative. Its sedative qualities make it ideal for treating such allergy symptoms as headaches, nausea, and depression. It can also be used as a mild analgesic to relieve overly tense muscles and body aches, and may be combined with thyme (an antispasmodic) and warming oils to soothe the aches and pains that come about as the result of a toxic body.

To make a lavender and herbal oil body rub mix ten drops of lavender oil with ten drops of thyme oil, five drops of juniper oil, ten drops of eucalyptus oil, five drops of pine oil, and four fluid ounces of almond or wheat germ oil. Mix the oils together in a dark glass bottle and shake well before using. This oil is to be used externally only—as a rub to massage away muscles' aches and pains. To use it, pour about a teaspoonful of the oil onto your palms and rub your hands together to warm the oil, then massage gently into the painful area. Use the solution twice a day. As with any herbal preparation, special care must be taken. Do not use it on or around the facial area, and discontinue use if a rash should develop. Do not use it if you are pregnant or suffer from high blood pressure, and reduce the dosage by half if you have sensitive skin. Note: Epileptics or those with nerve disorders should avoid using pine oil.

Ginger Root, Peppermint, and Chamomile Combined,

ginger root, peppermint, and chamomile make a great remedy for soothing an upset stomach. Once you've blended them, you might add one teaspoon of the mixture (you can use the commercially prepared dried form) to a cup of boiled water. Then steep for ten minutes before drinking.

Yoga   Yoga is a particularly good exercise for those who are dealing with all kinds of allergies, including reactions to environmental pollution, because it is holistic, based on the awareness of mind and body. Allergic reactions are often influenced by this mind-body interplay. Creating a sense of tranquillity with meditation and calming yoga postures supports the immune system.

One example of a yoga exercise that is relaxing and beneficial to allergy sufferers is the *corpse (Shavasana)* posture. It is an excellent relaxation technique that strengthens nervous-system functioning. It also benefits circulation and helps to reduce fatigue as well as relax the skeletal muscles. It is quite easy to do, even for the beginner or for those who are not in great shape. To begin, dim the lights and lie on your back—having placed a soft mat or towel on the floor first—spreading your arms about twelve to eighteen inches from your sides. Be sure that your palms are open and facing up, then spread your feet as wide as your shoulders. Place a folded towel behind your head and neck. Close your eyes. Breathe slowly and deeply, allowing the abdomen to rise and fall with each inhalation and exhalation. Practice this exercise for five to ten minutes. When the routine is completed, you should feel more relaxed, calmer, and ready for your complete yoga session.

For more information on yoga, a catalog of more than sixty books, audio cassettes and videos, as well as information on the locations of yoga centers throughout the country, contact the Himalayan Institute of Yoga, Science, and Philosophy, RRI Box 400, Honesdale, Pennsylvania 18431, or call (800) 822-4547.

Hydrotherapy An alternative health care provider might suggest hydrotherapy treatments to detoxify, energize, and cleanse the body. Since the start of civilization, water has been recognized for its therapeutic value. Water cleanses. That's why we need to drink enough water daily; in times of stress and illness, baths and compresses can effectively ease pain and cleanse the body of toxins.

There are many elaborate systems of hydrotherapy such as the ones that are used at health spas, but water's healing powers can also be utilized at home in the form of a soothing, old-fashioned bath. By adding commercially prepared herbs, oils, and minerals to your next tub of water, you can maximize the therapeutic effects of the bath. But always consult your primary health care provider before using any herb, particularly in the case of pregnant women, children, or people who have certain medical conditions or are using any medication. Do not use any herb for a prolonged period of time, combine herbs on your own, or use any herb in large doses. Some herbs can be toxic in small doses so never use a herb you are unfamiliar with or know little about. Be alert for any adverse reactions or side effects, which you should immediately discuss with your primary health care provider.

Depending on your particular symptoms, specific baths can be helpful in treating stress, relieving itchy and irritated skin, releasing toxins, and stimulating digestive processes. Water temperatures will vary according to your needs. Hot baths relax the body and stimulate the immune system. If they are hot enough to create perspiration, they facilitate detoxification. Cold baths work to reduce inflammation and fatigue. Here are some useful treatments:

- *Apple cider vinegar* is used in many folk recipes and is said to detoxify, combat fatigue, and restore the acid balance of the skin. Add one cup to a warm bath.
- *Sea salt* has been reported to detoxify the body; add one pound to hot water. For additional benefit, you might add one pound of baking soda.
- *Baking soda* relieves skin irritation and itch, and it aids in the release of toxins. Add two pounds to your bath.
- *Cornstarch* reportedly helps relieve the itching from skin irritation. Add one pound to your bath.

TREATMENTS FOR INDUSTRIAL AND INORGANIC ALLERGIES

Conventional	Alternative
Avoidance	**Hydrotherapy**
Eliminating allergens and using air filters	Specific baths for specific conditions
Staying away during toxic changes in workplace	
Wearing protective clothing	
Changing chemical or household products	
	Herbs
	Specific herbs for specific symptoms
	Massage
	Swedish, seaweed, self-massage, aromatherapy
	Yoga

Combined Treatments

When treating industrial and inorganic allergies, it is important that we draw from every healing source, whether it be allopathic or alternative. Proper testing to determine the precise causes of the allergies is extremely important, as is keeping a diary of symptoms. A thorough physical examination in the allopathic tradition is a good choice and excellent starting point. In all cases, removal and avoidance of the allergens, if possible and not impractical, is the best remedy. However, that is not always as effortless and practical to do as changing our household cleaners. We cannot escape from the pollution in our offices or the smog that chokes our highways. We can't hide from the toxic external world. Instead, we can build our immune systems, exercise, and meditate to relieve the stress and tension that weaken us, leaving us vulnerable to pollutants.

We can create a total treatment program by combining allopathic and alternative methods, for instance, by getting yearly physical examinations from an allopathic health care provider, removing allergens from our immediate environment, and treating ourselves to massage sessions and yoga classes to relieve stress. Additional steps that we can take and integrate into a total treatment program include: using natural housecleaning products and store-bought cleansers that remove chemicals from fruits and produce; wearing and using natural-fiber and dye-free organic clothing; growing chemical-free vegetables; and seeking out nontoxic places to live or homes built with environmental concerns in mind.

If you would like more information about additional measures you can take you can contact these valuable resources:

Chemical Injury Research
Foundation (CIRF)
3639 N. Pearl Street
Tacoma, WA 98407
(206) 752-6677

Environmental Health Letter
P.O. Box 3638
Syracuse, NY 13220
(315) 455-7862

CHAPTER 9

Juvenile Allergies

For the majority of people, allergies begin in infancy or childhood. Parents raising an allergic child are faced with the difficulty of handling a child who can turn from delightful to cranky and teary-eyed in the blink of an eye. Add a runny nose, sneezing, itchy skin, and a rash, and you get a not-quite-so-pleasant picture.

All parents want their children to be happy and healthy. During times of impaired health, parental support is more important than ever to accomplish such goals. When children are suffering from allergies, not only are they physically ill, but they are probably angry and upset about it. After all, if life is fair, why can't Susie or Jimmy play in the grass and not break out in hives? Coping with your child's allergies isn't going to be easy, but there are enough treatment options to make it less difficult. Understanding the roots of allergies and why they affect your child in particular ways is a major step toward helping your child live comfortably with the condition. Since allergies affect infants and children in different ways than they affect adults, this chapter will offer solutions that are tailored exclusively for them. After reading this chapter you will feel more confident about having the necessary tools to help your child play, sleep, and generally spend the day more comfortably. There is no cure for allergies, but there are ways to make the symptoms almost disappear.

EXPLORING THE ROOTS OF JUVENILE ALLERGIES

Allergic disorders have the dubious distinction of ranking first among children's chronic diseases. Allergies start early. Infants often develop allergic reactions to milk that result in bloody diarrhea, weight loss, and other symptoms. Cradle cap—the scaling of the skin on an infant's scalp—is a form of allergy, often referred to as atopic dermatitis. Sniffles, coughs, and diaper rashes can all be caused by allergies.

Children have immune systems that are still developing and that are much more sensitive to illness and less effective than adult systems in fighting it off. Their skin is also more fragile than that of adults. It is important to recognize and treat the symptoms of allergy in order to minimize the damage from repeated assaults on the immune system and other body functions.

Although some of the following symptoms may have a variety of causes, your child may suffer from allergies if you notice:

* itchy, watery eyes
* dark circles under the eyes that resemble "shiners"
* recurrent sinus or ear infections
* watery, clear nasal discharge
* breathing from the mouth and frequent clearing of the throat
* rashes on the skin, hives, eczema
* a chronic cough, wheezing, and/or chest congestion
* diarrhea, bloating, gas, nausea, vomiting

- symptoms that recur seasonally
- hyperactive behavior, temper tantrums, irritability

There are many types of allergies, and we are going to touch on the most common in this chapter. We suggest that you also read chapter 1, "Introduction to Asthma, Allergies, and Food Sensitivities," for a more comprehensive view of what allergies are about, as well as the chapters on juvenile asthma; food allergies; skin allergies and eczema; and hay fever and allergic rhinitis. The topic of allergies is very complex and requires a broad range of theories and factors to fully explain or explore it. What we have done in this chapter is to condense the vast amount of research, theory, and clinical insights on allergy as it applies particularly to infants and children and their unique treatment needs.

MILK ALLERGY AND LACTOSE INTOLERANCE

Milk is a common allergen in children and in infants. Symptoms are severe in infants, often taking the form of diarrhea, rashes, asthma, and a variety of infections worrisome enough to give parents some sleepless nights. Since milk allergies in infants are a serious problem, a physician should be consulted at once. A number of factors contribute to an infant's developing an allergy to milk. They include: heredity; introduction to solid foods too early; and being fed cow's milk rather than breast milk, which may prevent the infant from developing the necessary antibodies.

Sometimes what is thought to be a milk allergy is actually lactose intolerance, which can be determined by many tests. One test measures the pH level in a fresh stool sample to determine whether or not glucose is present and the stool is acidic. An acidic stool is an indicator of lactose intolerance.

For further information about lactose intolerance, refer to the chapter on food sensitivities in this book.

SKIN ALLERGIES

Skin rashes and irritations have a variety of causes. Ironically, some medications that are supposed to cure us—such as penicillin, sulfur, insulin, and antibiotics—may actually cause hives, the itchy, raised bumps that may appear suddenly and just as suddenly disappear. Other causes for this reaction may be allergens, such as food additives or foods, including berries, nuts, and chocolate, among others. Hives may also appear after exposure to certain plants, insect bites, pollen, injections, changes in temperature, and chemicals. In acute cases, hives may result in severe allergic reactions, such as anaphylaxis, which can interfere with breathing or swallowing. Get emergency help immediately.

ALLERGIC RHINITIS AND HAY FEVER

Children suffering from allergic rhinitis or hay fever tend to develop a recognizable look; that is, they tend to have dark circles around their eyes; and, because they wipe their noses often and vigorously, there may be a crease between the tip and bridge of the nose. You'll notice sneezing and sometimes a buck-toothed expression that comes from prying open their mouths with their fingers in order to breathe more easily.

There are two main inhalant allergies that could be making your child miserable. Allergic rhinitis can be seasonal (occurring in the spring and fall), due to exposure to pollens, grasses, or weeds; hay fever is caused by seasonal pollens such as the infamous ragweed plant. On the other hand, perennial allergic rhinitis occurs with exposure to indoor allergens such as pet dander, dust mites, and other offenders. These two allergies spring from different causes, but they are equally annoying.

Allergies should never be ignored in the hope that they will go away. Allergy symptoms such as mouth breathing have serious long-term implications. The continuous air pressure it causes can change the way that the soft bones of your child's face grow, abnormally elongating the face and forcing the teeth to come in at incorrect angles. This will create dental problems, such as an overbite, and your child may need braces as a result. Chronic dental problems such as tooth decay are another side effect of untreated allergies. Ear infections that are chronic and untreated can lead to hearing loss, which can lead to poor grades, loss of confidence, and poor speech. Toddlers and small children with runny noses often stuff their noses with tissues, which can result in a discharge from the affected nostril. Untreated allergies can interfere with normal childhood activities and leave your child feeling a bit like a wallflower. These are just some of the reasons why it is so important to take your child to a physician or allergist as soon as allergies are suspected.

FOOD ALLERGY

You can't fool Mother Nature, especially when it comes to feeding your newborn infant; mother's milk is the perfect food for a newborn infant, and in the interest of protecting your child from allergies it is advisable to breast-feed for the first year if possible. Mothers who are breast-feeding should avoid foods that are likely to cause allergic reactions. Try not to eat milk, eggs, peanuts, fish, citrus fruits, wheat, beef, and chicken—or any food to which your other children may be allergic, since your infant may have the same allergies. As the infant grows, it is best to feed him foods such as carrots, pears, rice, and lamb, for example, that generally don't cause allergic reactions in adults. Avoid foods—particularly wheat, eggs, corn products, citrus fruits, sugar, and chocolate—which are known to cause allergic reactions, until the infant's system is more developed. Solid foods should be introduced slowly and in small quantities. Observe your child to see if there are any adverse reactions to foods as they are introduced into the diet. As the child becomes accustomed to a variety of foods that do not commonly cause allergies, foods such as wheat and eggs (after the child is about a year old) can be introduced.

Food allergies play a major role in childhood asthma and hay fever. Common allergens are milk, nuts, eggs, fish, shell-fish, nuts, and peanuts, as well as food colorings. The sooner allergies are caught and treated, the better for your child's general health and well-being. If you suspect allergies, take your child to a physician or allergist to be tested and treated. A severe reaction to a food allergen—peanuts, for example—can lead to anaphylactic shock, which is life threatening.

Infants and young children usually don't miss the foods that they are allergic to, but older children who suffer from food allergies often feel deprived. The truth is that most people crave the foods they're allergic to, and kids are no different. Try to make the new diet as much fun as possible, and offer substitute foods that taste good. Eventually your children will learn to love the foods that are good for them and will lose their taste for the food that they cannot tolerate. When you first withdraw problem foods, however, there will be a difficult period of physical and mental withdrawal that may include sulking and temper tantrums. Explain to your children that they will feel better and be able to play longer and harder if they stick to the foods you are giving them. Once they begin to feel healthier and their allergy symptoms are reduced, the children will realize that you are telling the truth. And after all, no one wants to return to a stuffy nose, headache, and other allergy symptoms.

Traditional Treatments

If you suspect that your child may suffer from allergies, go either to your primary health care provider or to a physician whose specialty is juvenile allergies. Once you have identified the offending allergens, you can take measures to remove or eliminate them from your child's environment or diet. Skin testing for allergies is preferable to blood tests—although, in the case of food allergies, it is possible to have a positive test to food that is not causing symptoms. Changes in diet should not be based on skin tests alone, but on a combination of tests and other evaluations. If a skin test for food allergies is positive, the next diagnostic step should be a double-blind challenge to make sure that the diagnosis is correct. Many health care providers, both traditional and alternative, will prescribe some form of the elimination diet to test for food allergies. See chapter 6 for a detailed discussion of the elimination diet.

If environmental factors, such as dust mites, mold, or pet dander, are a problem, you should make sure that your child's teacher and school nurse are aware of the situation. Some environmental allergies are easier to control than others. You simply take small and common-sense measures, such as having your child sit away from the blackboard if there is a sensitivity to chalk dust, or having your child take a bath before bedtime to avoid bringing allergens into bed. At home, you can remove feathers, down, carpets, heavy drapes, pets, and even stuffed animals from your child's bedroom, since these are favored haunts of the dust mite.

Clean and vacuum closets regularly, disinfect your bathroom, and keep your home well ventilated in order to make it less hospitable to mold. Additional measures that you can take to rid your child's environment of allergens are outlined in chapter 3, on juvenile asthma, of this book.

Medications

In the allopathic medical tradition, your child's allergy symptoms will be treated with various medications. Children are somewhat more limited here than adults, since adult allergy medications are not suitable for use by children. However, there are certainly enough medications available, prescription and nonprescription, to treat symptoms such as chest congestion, skin rashes, hives, runny noses, and watery eyes. When taking any medication, your child should always be observed closely to see if an unusual reaction occurs. Nasal sprays can be addicting and are often overused, which results in a "rebound" effect that clogs the nose and puts you right back where you started. If your child uses a medicated nasal spray, you might buy a bottle of saline nasal mist for occasional use to soothe the delicate nasal membranes, which can get irritated from the overuse of nasal sprays and decongestants.

Following is a list of the most commonly used medications for children:

Corticosteroid Nasal Sprays   Prescribed for children (age six or older) to reduce inflammation in the nasal passages caused by hay fever and allergic rhinitis, corticosteroid nasal sprays work to relieve the symptoms of congestion, sneezing, runny nose and itching. Beclomethasone products (Vancenase and Beconase AQ) are the only nasal sprays approved for children as young as six years of age. They can also be used by adults.

Nasal Corticosteroids Not to be confused with anabolic steroids, the drugs used by some athletes to build muscle and bulk, nasal corticosteroids have been found to be safe and effective, although some patients do experience side effects, such as sneezing, irritation of the nose, dryness, and nosebleeds. In the case of hives that do not respond to treatment with antihistamines, many physicians will prescribe corticosteroid drugs to be used in conjunction with the antihistamines.

Antihistamines Antihistamines work to reduce the action of histamines, which are produced when your child inhales pollen, dust, mold, or other inhalants. They are most effective in treating such allergy symptoms as itchy, watery eyes, runny nose, sneezing, and other symptoms of hay fever and allergic rhinitis. Nonprescription antihistamines can have unpleasant side effects, however, such as drowsiness, dizziness, and dry mouth. If your child is using antihistamines, you should notify the child's teacher and ask to be contacted if your child has trouble concentrating or participating in school activities. Nonsedating antihistamines are available by prescription for children age twelve and older, and they can be a good alternative medication for older children who wish to avoid the side effects of over-the-counter antihistamines.

Cromolyn Sodium Nasal Sprays A cromolyn sodium nasal spray, such as Nasalcrom®, is often used to prevent nasal inflammation that results in congestion. Although side effects are very rare, some people experience side effects that include sneezing, a burning sensation in the nose, nasal irritation, and headache. If your child shows any of these symptoms while using the spray, stop using it at once.

Hydrocortisone Applied topically for its anti-inflammatory qualities, hydrocortisone is used to treat skin allergies such as eczema.

Decongestants Taken by mouth or applied locally through nasal sprays or drops, decongestants are often prescribed to eliminate the nasal congestion caused by allergies.

Immunotherapy (Allergy Shots) This process of allergy injection is a long-term commitment not generally advised for most people. If you feel that your child's allergy symptoms cannot be controlled by changes in the environment or medication, then this might be a last-resort option. Refer to the discussion of immunotherapy in the adult asthma chapter for more details.

Alternative Treatments Selecting alternative treatments for your child's allergies is a difficult task. You want to do the best thing for your child, and you're pulled in many directions. The allopathic medical world will tell you that without proper treatment and medication—cortisone, antihistamines, and decongestants—your child's allergies will not only fail to get better but they will eventually get worse. On the other hand the natural, chemical-free appeal of alternative remedies may seem like a "kinder, gentler" approach. What should you do?

First and foremost, your child should see an allopathic physician for the initial allergy treatment. There are many reasons for this recommendation, not least of which is the necessity of diagnosing the presence of life-threatening allergic reactions known as anaphylactic shock. Once you have a prescribed (medically approved) diagnosis and treatment plan in hand, you may begin to discuss alternative options with your primary health care provider. Your pediatrician or allergist can help you choose treatments that will not react or interfere with the basic therapies he or she is administering. Most people don't realize it, but even the seemingly benign practice of adding vitamins to your diet can interfere with prescribed medications or other medical treatment. However, you probably will find a way to integrate natural and allopathic treatments if you and your doctor work together toward that goal. Having witnessed the long-term futility of overprescribing antibiotics and other medications for colds and infections, more and more allopathic health care providers are open to discussing natural therapies in an overall allergy treatment plan.

Herbal Treatments

Herbs can be used to relieve various conditions—for instance, nasal congestion, nausea, and diarrhea—stemming from food allergies; they can also ease the itch and irritation resulting from hives and other skin allergies. Children need to take special precautions when being treated with herbs because their other organs and skin are more fragile than adults', and remedies must be tailored to their special needs.

Following are some general guidelines:

- Herbs should be greatly diluted for children, who should never be given adult doses.
- Always consult your pediatrician about any herbal treatment you plan on administering. It is also advisable to consult with an herbal practitioner who has experience in prescribing for children.
- Never give your child a remedy that he or she finds distasteful or upsetting.
- Always observe your child after administering a remedy. Be on the alert for any negative reactions.
- Look for signs that the remedy is working. Not all remedies are appropriate for every child.
- If your child's condition worsens, discontinue use and seek medical attention.

- Educate yourself about the use of herbs. Learn about their specific characteristics, possible toxic side effects, and proper dosages. Become aware of how herbs interact with each other, with various foods, and with allopathic medications. Refer to the Appendix at the back of this book for the names of organizations offering information about herbs.

- If your child is taking an herb on a daily basis, refrain from using it for at least one week during the month so that your child does not build a resistance to it. Herbs lose their effectiveness if they are used excessively.

- Never use herbs found in the wild. Always purchase your herbs from a reputable store.

Some herbal remedies are described below. Check with your doctor to make sure they are appropriate for your child.

Ginger* Ginger is a warm herb that has been used as a tonic for centuries. It can safely reduce the symptoms of food allergy, such as indigestion, nausea, and gas. To make the perfect cup of ginger tea, put cold tap water into a kettle and bring it to a boil. Measure one teaspoon of commercially prepared dried ginger root into one cup of water, let steep for five minutes, and then strain into a mug. Serve several times a day or until symptoms are relieved.

Calendula (Pot Marigold) Often sold in creams for external use on skin allergies such as eczema, Calendula (also known as pot marigold) has anti-inflammatory effects.

Comfrey Comfrey can be used in salve form to cover skin inflammations such as eczema. You can find comfrey salves ready-made in health food stores.

---

*Ginger is not recommended for use by children under three years of age.

Burdock The leaves, roots, and seeds of the burdock are used for various treatments, including topical applications that heal skin eruptions, psoriasis, and eczema.

Diet and Nutrition

Alternative health care providers believe that the causes of systemic allergies almost always result from the diet. Allergies may be linked to pollens and other allergens in the environment, but they would never develop if foods that offend the immune system were not eaten. In other words, the problem dates back to the initial feeding process, usually with the introduction of cow's milk, formula, and solid foods before the digestive system has matured. Food allergens are thus introduced into fragile systems that are simply not equipped to handle these substances, and allergic reactions may develop in response.

Alternative health care providers base their treatment of allergies on their suspicion of food allergy as the underlying cause. Given this basic premise, the alternative practitioner diagnoses and treats juvenile allergies with special diets, nutritional and vitamin supplements, and herbs. An elimination diet is based on foods not likely to cause an allergic reaction in the child (see the discussion of food allergies in chapter 6 for step-by-step instructions). As toxins are removed from the child's system by adherence to this diet, additional foods are reintroduced after a week or more. If an allergic reaction occurs, the new food is quickly withdrawn.

An alternative health care provider may also prescribe a rotation, or "rotary," diet (see chapter 6 for details) to treat food allergies. The theory behind such a diet is that lessening exposure to known allergies will prevent new allergies from forming. Foods that are tolerated are eaten once every four to seven days, giving the body time to clear out antibodies that may create symptoms. Foods that have been eliminated for a period of time can gradually be reintroduced. This diet involves a great deal of planning, and you may even require a nutritionist to help design it. Although once a rotation pattern has been established, it becomes easier to plan a menu around the diet, it does take time and effort to make it work. Additional dietary measures may be necessary to clear up skin allergies, and the consumption of essential fatty acids found in salmon, tuna, and other fatty fish are often recommended.

Homeopathy

Most homeopathic physicians will recommend finding the source of an allergy and then avoiding it or removing it until symptoms clear up. However, there are times when they will provide custom remedies to combat the symptoms and treat the underlying systemic imbalances. A homeopath who mixes a combination remedy to relieve a broad range of symptoms—sneezing, headaches, watery eyes—assumes that the body will assimilate what it needs to heal and reject what it doesn't. Because homeopaths treat each case as unique, remedies are usually based on extensive evaluation of factors such as symptoms, lifestyle, stress levels, and environment. Standard formulas are not simply doled out as a matter of course, but rather are carefully concocted to treat individual needs.

Some typical homeopathic allergy remedies that may be given to children include the following:

- *Pulsitilla:* used for treating allergies and ear infections when the child is tearful and upset

- *Sabadilla:* a common remedy for symptoms of allergic rhinitis and hay fever, such as runny nose, sneezing, and itchy, watery eyes
- *Wyethia:* used to treat a runny nose, and dryness in the throat and nasal passages
- *Arsenicum album:* used to treat allergic symptoms such as a runny nose, headaches, and coughing as well as asthma
- *Chamomila:* used to calm irritable, fussy children
- *Apis:* demonstrating quite clearly that what can kill you can also cure you, this remedy contains a substance derived from bee venom—effective on very itchy hives worsened by exposure to warmth or changes in the weather
- *Anacardium:* used for symptoms such as blisters filled with yellow fluid

TREATMENTS FOR JUVENILE ALLERGIES

Conventional	Alternative
Environmental Changes	*Environmental Changes*
Removal of allergens from diet and environment	Removal of allergens
Immunotherapy (Allergy shots)	
Medications	*Diet and Nutrition*
Corticosteroid nasal sprays, antihistamines, hydrocortisone	Removal of food allergens, rotation diet, elimination diet
	Herbal Treatments

Combined Treatments

As we have mentioned, juvenile allergies should always be treated by a medical doctor. There is no question that allopathic treatment plays a vital role in treating allergies, particularly in severe and acute cases. First, allergies must be identified through medical tests. Then, it is best to avoid or eliminate allergens from your child's environment and life. After those two vital steps have been taken, however, alternative therapies can be implemented to assist in healing.

The best way to treat allergies in the first place is to begin a program of allergy prevention in the infant's early years. When pregnant, try to avoid eating large amounts of foods that can be passed on to the child as allergens, such as chocolate or peanuts. Breast-feed your baby to boost the fragile immune system, which is so susceptible to allergens. Don't introduce solid foods into the diet before your infant is mature enough for them.

Your child's allopathic program can include prescription or nonprescription medication to relieve symptoms, avoidance of the allergen and, if everything else has failed, allergy shots. You can turn to alternative medicine to complement such treatments. For example, your child may have been using a nonprescription nasal spray to relieve congestion. In order to avoid the "rebound" effect that is caused by overuse and oversensitivity to the medication itself, you might want to alternate it with use of an herbal tea suited for relieving congestion.

Here are some other suggestions for adding allopathic or alternative therapies to your child's treatment program:

- In place of hydrocortisone, which can thin the skin if overused, use herbal skin creams such as comfrey, burdock, and marigold for external treatment of skin irritations.

- To complement an allopathic treatment program, meet with a homeopath to discuss homeopathic remedies for treating allergy symptoms such as runny noses and itching.
- Work with a nutritionist to design a healthy, allergen-free diet for your child.
- Use bodywork to relieve your child's allergic symptoms and reduce the stress of living with allergies.
- Alternate commercially prepared herbal teas with antacids to relieve upset stomach and gas that accompany food allergies. For allergies such as hay fever, consider using homeopathic nasal sprays (such as Similasan Nasal Spray) sold in health-food stores as an alternative to chemical sprays, thus avoiding the "rebound" effect.
- Supplement your child's diet with nutritional supplements, such as evening primrose capsules, to treat skin allergies. Good nutrition is a firm foundation for any medical plan.
- Learn more about alternative therapies that may be beneficial for your child. If one treatment does not work, don't be afraid to explore related options. For example, if you take your child for an acupressure massage and your child doesn't like it, you might try a Swedish massage the next time, or ask the practitioner to recommend another type of bodywork that will suit your child's needs.
- Enjoy learning more about health care and make it fun for your child too. A good attitude is an essential part of any medical program, so don't let anxiety about your child's condition rub off on your child. Smile!

Appendix: Resources and Organizations

Acupressure Institute
1533 Shattuck Avenue
Berkeley, CA 94709
(510) 845-1059

Allergy Information
 Association
65 Tromley Drive, Suite 10
Etobicoke, Ont. M9B5Y7,
 Canada

Allergy Publications
P.O. Box 640
Menlo Park, CA 94026

American Academy of
 Allergy and Immunology
611 E. Wells Street
Milwaukee, WI 53202
(800) 822-ASMA

American Allergy
 Association
P.O. Box 7273
Menlo Park, CA 94026
(415) 322-1663

American Association of
 Acupuncture and Oriental
 Medicine
433 Front Street
Cataswqua, PA 18032
(610) 433-2448

American Association of
 Oriental Healing Arts
P.O. Box 718
Jamaica Plains, MA 02130
(617) 236-5867

American Botanical Council
P.O. Box 201660
Austin, TX 78720
(512) 331-8868

American Chiropractic
 Association
1701 Clarendon Boulevard
Arlington, VA 22209
(703) 276-8800

American Herbal Products
 Association
4733 Bethesda Avenue,
 Suite 345
Bethesda, MD 20814
(301) 951-3204

American Holistic Medical
 Association
2727 Fairview Avenue East,
 Suite B
Seattle, WA 98102
(206) 322-6842

American Massage Therapy
Association
820 Davis Street, Suite 100
Evanston, IL 60201
(312) 761-2682

American Osteopathic
Association
142 East Ontario Street
Chicago, IL 60611
(312) 280-5800

American Yoga Association
P.O. Box 18105
Cleveland Heights, OH
44118
(216) 371-0078

Asthma and Allergy
Foundation of America
1125 15th Street NW Suite
502
Washington, D.C. 20005
(800) 7-ASTHMA

Center for Medical
Consumers
237 Thompson Street
New York, NY 10012
(212) 674-7105

Centers for Disease Control
and Prevention
4770 Buford Highway NE
Atlanta, GA 30341-3724
(800) 488-7330

Chemical Injury Research
Foundation (CIRF)
3639 N. Pearl Street
Tacoma, WA 98407
(206) 752-6677

Eczema Association
1221 SW Yamhill, Suite 303
Portland, OR 97205
(503) 228-4430

Environmental Health Letter
P.O. Box 3638
Syracuse, NY 13220
(315) 455-7862

Environmental Protection
Agency (EPA)
Indoor Air Quality
Clearinghouse
P.O. Box 37133
Washington, D.C. 20013
(800) 438-4319

Food Allergy Network
4744 Holly Avenue
Fairfax, VA 22030
(800) 929-4040

Food and Drug
Administration (FDA)
Rockville, MD 20857
(301) 443-3170

The Herb Research
Foundation
1007 Pearl Street, Suite 200
Boulder, CO 80830
(303) 449-2265

Institute of Rehabilitative
Nutrition
P.O. Box 20199
Columbus Circle Station
New York, NY 10023
(800) 839-6554

International Academy of
Nutritional Medicine
P.O. Box 5832
Lincoln, NE 68505
(402) 467-2716

International Foundation for
Homeopathy
2366 Eastlake Avenue East,
Suite 301
Seattle, WA 98102
(206) 324-8230

International Institute of
Reflexology
P.O. Box 12462
St. Petersburg, FL 33733
(813) 343-4811

Medic Alert
2323 Colorado Avenue
Turlock, CA 95382
(209) 668-3333

Mothers of Asthmatics
3554 Chain Bridge Road
Suite 200
Fairfax, VA 22030-2709
(800) 878-4403

National Commission for the
Certification of
Acupuncturists
1424 16 Street NW, Suite 501
Washington, D.C. 20036
(202) 232-1404

National Digestive Diseases
Information Clearinghouse
(for materials on lactose
intolerance)
(301) 468-6344

National Institute of Allergy
and Infectious Diseases
9000 Rockville Pike
Bethesda, MD 20892
(301) 496-2563

National Jewish Center for
Immunology and
Respiratory Medicine
1400 Jackson Street
Denver, CO 80206
(800) 222-LUNG

Natural Lifestyle Supplies
16 Lookout Drive
Asheville, NC
(704) 254-9606
(products for people
suffering from
environmental illnesses)

Office of Alternative
Medicine
NIH Information Center,
Suite 450
Rockville, MD 20852
(301) 402-2466

Transcendental Meditation
P.O. Box 49667
Colorado Springs, CO
80949-9667
(800) 843-8332

Glossary

Acupressure The technique, taken from Oriental medicine, of applying pressure on specific body points to restore energy and balance, promote relaxation, and improve circulation.

Acupuncture The technique, based in Oriental medicine, of inserting needles into specific body points to relieve disease symptoms.

Acute Used to describe an episode of intense illness or reaction that requires emergency medical care.

Additives Substances, such as preservatives, that are added to foods to preserve freshness or to enhance their appearance, taste, color, and smell.

Adrenaline A hormone secreted by the adrenal glands. Its injectible form is epinephrine, which is used to treat severe allergic reactions and asthma attacks.

Airways The air passages extending from the nose to the lungs. *See* bronchi.

Allergen A substance that causes an allergic response.

Allergy An altered or exaggerated susceptibility to various foreign substances or physical agents.

Anaphylaxis, or Anaphylactic Shock A severe allergic reaction that can result in death. Major symptoms include difficulty in breathing and swallowing, as well as hives.

Antacid A substance used to reduce excess acidity of the stomach contents.

Antibodies Proteins produced by the immune system in response to the introduction of foreign proteins, including allergens.

Antigen Any substance that, under favorable conditions, can stimulate the production of antibodies.

Antihistamine A drug used to treat allergic reactions by counteracting the effects of histamine, which cause allergy and asthma symptoms.

Anti-Inflammatory A substance that soothes and reduces inflammation.

Asthma An obstruction of the bronchial tubes characterized by wheezing and difficulty in breathing, coughing, and chest constriction.

Bronchi The two main airways connected and leading up to the lungs.

Bronchodilator A medication used by asthmatics to open constricted airways.

Candidiasis An infection caused by an overgrowth of the yeastlike fungi normally found in the body.

Challenge Testing A method of determining allergic sensitivity by exposure to a suspected substance and observations of a reaction.

Chi (also spelled *qui*) In Oriental medicine and acupuncture, the vital life energy which courses through the body.

Chronic The opposite of acute, used to describe a disease or illness of long duration, marked by recurring episodes.

Contact Dermatitis An allergic skin irritation or rash that results from direct contact with specific allergens.

Corticosteroids A family of potent hormones used therapeutically to treat inflammatory and allergic disorders. Also called steroids.

Dander Tiny particles of an animal's skin or hair that frequently cause allergic reactions.

Decongestant A drug used to shrink swollen membranes and blood vessels, particularly in the nasal and sinus area.

Eczema An itchy, dry, scaly rash. Some authorities limit the word "eczema" to cases springing from internal causes and call those caused by external contact "dermatitis" or "eczematous dermatitis."

Elimination Diet A diet that eliminates commonly allergenic foods, or temporarily avoids foods suspected of causing allergies, in order to pinpoint food allergens in affected individuals.

Epinephrine The adrenal hormone that is injected to treat anaphylactic shock.

Essential Oils The concentrated oils extracted from a plant's flower, leaves, branches, or roots. Most often used in baths, massage treatments, and aromatherapy.

Expectorant A drug or herbal remedy that promotes the loosening and expulsion of phlegm from the lungs.

FDA The Food and Drug Administration, a government regulatory agency that oversees food and drug safety, and approves the use and sale of new pharmaceuticals and medications.

Hay Fever A seasonal allergic reaction to pollen.

Herbalism The practice of using herbal remedies to treat illness and to preserve and restore health.

Histamine A naturally occurring chemical substance in body tissues. When histamine is overproduced in an allergy, it results in allergy symptoms.

Hives Itchy, red welts that accompany an allergic reaction; also known as urticaria.

Holistic Used to describe a preventative approach to health and medicine that treats the entire individual, emphasizing the interdependence of the mind and body.

Homeopathy A holistic method of treating disease, based on the theory that a substance causing disease in a healthy person may also cure the disease; homeopaths prepare natural remedies tailored to each patient.

IgE (immunoglobulin E) The antibody that is most frequently involved in immediate allergic reactions. Produced by the immune system in response to an allergen, it results in symptoms of allergy such as sneezing, flushing, congestion, and other signs.

Immune System The mechanism the body uses to resist disease, producing antibodies that neutralize, metabolize, or eliminate antigens.

Immunotherapy The process of boosting the body's resistance to an allergen by repeated exposure to a diluted version of the offending substance.

Inflammation The body's response to injury, irritants, or infection with pain, heat, or swelling.

Inhalant Microscopic airborne particles, such as dust, dander, or mold, that provoke an allergic reaction when inhaled.

Irritant Any substance that causes local irritation.

Lactase An intestinal enzyme that converts milk sugar (lactose) into glucose and galactose; a deficiency of this enzyme causes lactose intolerance.

Lactose Sugar derived from milk and dairy products; lactose intolerance is the inability to digest lactose.

Mast cells Cells containing histamine found in the mucous membranes, skin, and bronchial tubes.

Meridian According to Oriental medicine, one of the fourteen channels in the body through which the *chi* (life force) flows. *See also* chi.

Mite A microscopic insect that feeds on human and animal skin and feathers. Often found in rugs, pillows, carpeting, bedding, and dust, mites are common allergens.

Mold A multicellular fungus that causes an allergic reaction in sensitive individuals when inhaled.

Mucus The thick fluid secreted by the mucous membranes.

Nasal Polyps Growths in the nose that can block the nasal passages and are sometimes related to allergies.

Over-the-Counter (OTC) Drugs Medications that have FDA approval to be sold without a prescription.

Peak Expiratory Flow Rate The maximum rate at which air can be exhaled.

Peak Flow Meter Hand-held device that is used to measure peak expiratory flow in order to predict and prevent an asthma attack.

Pollen Microscopic spores from grasses, flowers, and trees that may cause hay fever and other allergies when inhaled.

Rebound Effect The flare-up of allergic symptoms that occurs when a medicine that one has been taking regularly is withdrawn.

Rotation Diet A diet in which different foods are rotated to avoid frequent exposure to known allergens and to prevent new allergies from developing. Foods are eaten once every four to seven days and gradually reintroduced into the diet; also known as a rotary diet.

Sinusitis A bacterial infection of the sinus cavities.

Skin Test An allergy test conducted by scratching or pricking the skin and then applying the suspected allergen.

Theophylline A bronchodilator, or medication used to clear the airways that are constricted in asthma.

Therapy In the context of the allopathic or alternative treatments, a program for relieving symptoms and healing medical disorders.

Urticaria Allergic hives or welts.

Wheal A raised area of skin that is measured to determine allergic sensitivity.

Yin/Yang A Chinese concept describing all existence in terms of conditions that are different but mutually dependent. In a healthy individual, yin and yang exist in a perpetually balanced state.

Index

Index to Allopathic Treatments